Objectively Structured Clinical Examination (OSCE) in Ophthalmology

Objectively Structured Clinical Examination (OSCE) in Ophthalmology

Second Edition

Editors

Amar Agarwal MS FRCS FRCOphth
Dr Agarwal's Group of Eye Hospitals and
Eye Research Centre
19 Cathedral Road, Chennai-600 086, Tamil Nadu, India

Dimple Prakash MS
Dr Agarwal's Group of Eye Hospitals and
Eye Research Centre
19 Cathedral Road, Chennai-600 086, Tamil Nadu, India

Athiya Agarwal MD FRSH DO
Dr Agarwal's Group of Eye Hospitals and
Eye Research Centre
19 Cathedral Road, Chennai-600 086, Tamil Nadu, India

Foreword
Kevin M Miller

JAYPEE BROTHERS MEDICAL PUBLISHERS (P) LTD

New Delhi • Ahmedabad • Bengaluru • Chennai • Hyderabad
Kochi • Kolkata • Lucknow • Mumbai Nagpur • St Louis (USA)

Published by
Jitendar P Vij
Jaypee Brothers Medical Publishers (P) Ltd
Corporate Office
4838/24 Ansari Road, Daryaganj, **New Delhi** - 110002, India, Phone: +91-11-43574357
Registered Office
B-3 EMCA House, 23/23B Ansari Road, Daryaganj, **New Delhi** - 110 002, India
Phones: +91-11-23272143, +91-11-23272703, +91-11-23282021
+91-11-23245672, Rel: +91-11-32558559, Fax: +91-11-23276490, +91-11-23245683
e-mail: jaypee@jaypeebrothers.com, Website: www.jaypeebrothers.com

Branches

- 2/B, Akruti Society, Jodhpur Gam Road Satellite
  Ahmedabad 380 015, Phones: +91-79-26926233, Rel: +91-79-32988717
  Fax: +91-79-26927094, e-mail: ahmedabad@jaypeebrothers.com

- 202 Batavia Chambers, 8 Kumara Krupa Road, Kumara Park East
  Bengaluru 560 001, Phones: +91-80-22285971, +91-80-22382956, 91-80-22372664
  Rel: +91-80-32714073, Fax: +91-80-22281761   e-mail: bangalore@jaypeebrothers.com

- 282 IIIrd Floor, Khaleel Shirazi Estate, Fountain Plaza, Pantheon Road
  Chennai 600 008, Phones: +91-44-28193265, +91-44-28194897, Rel: +91-44-32972089
   Fax: +91-44-28193231   e-mail: chennai@jaypeebrothers.com

- 4-2-1067/1-3, 1st Floor, Balaji Building, Ramkote Cross Road,
  Hyderabad 500 095, Phones: +91-40-66610020, +91-40-24758498
  Rel:+91-40-32940929, Fax:+91-40-24758499   e-mail: hyderabad@jaypeebrothers.com

- No. 41/3098, B & B1, Kuruvi Building, St. Vincent Road
  Kochi 682 018, Kerala, Phones: +91-484-4036109, +91-484-2395739
  +91-484-2395740   e-mail: kochi@jaypeebrothers.com

- 1-A Indian Mirror Street, Wellington Square
  Kolkata 700 013, Phones: +91-33-22651926, +91-33-22276404
  +91-33-22276415, Rel: +91-33-32901926, Fax: +91-33-22656075
  e-mail: kolkata@jaypeebrothers.com

- Lekhraj Market III, B-2, Sector-4, Faizabad Road, Indira Nagar
  Lucknow 226 016   Phones: +91-522-3040553, +91-522-3040554
  e-mail: lucknow@jaypeebrothers.com

- 106 Amit Industrial Estate, 61 Dr SS Rao Road, Near MGM Hospital, Parel
  Mumbai 400 012, Phones: +91-22-24124863, +91-22-24104532,
  Rel: +91-22-32926896, Fax: +91-22-24160828
  e-mail: mumbai@jaypeebrothers.com

- íKAMALPUSHPAî 38, Reshimbag, Opp. Mohota Science College, Umred Road
  Nagpur 440 009 (MS), Phone: Rel: +91-712-3245220, Fax: +91-712-2704275
  e-mail: nagpur@jaypeebrothers.com

USA Office
1745, Pheasant Run Drive, Maryland Heights (Missouri), MO 63043, USA, Ph: 001-636-6279734
e-mail: jaypee@jaypeebrothers.com, anjulav@jaypeebrothers.com

OSCE in Ophthalmology

© 2009, Amar Agarwal, Dimple Prakash, Athiya Agarwal

All rights reserved. No part of this publication should be reproduced, stored in a retrieval system, or transmitted in any form or by any means: electronic, mechanical, photocopying, recording, or otherwise, without the prior written permission of the editors and the publisher.

> This book has been published in good faith that the material provided by editors is original. Every effort is made to ensure accuracy of material, but the publisher, printer and editors will not be held responsible for any inadvertent error(s). In case of any dispute, all legal matters are to be settled under Delhi jurisdiction only.

First Edition: 2005

Second Edition: **2009**

ISBN 978-81-8448-612-4

Typeset at JPBMP typesetting unit
Printed at Sanat Printers, Kundli

*This book is dedicated to
Thomas Kohnen*

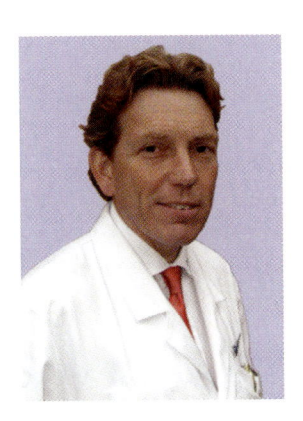

Foreword to the Second Edition

For decades, the assessment of cognitive knowledge and the evaluation of a medical doctor's ability to make appropriate medical decisions have been the responsibility of licensing agencies around the world. Once certified, it was usually expected that a practitioner would maintain competency through a self-directed course of continuing education. Traditionally, this was accomplished by requirement that license holders acquire a certain number of continuing medical education credits over a multi-year cycle by taking courses offered by accredited medical schools and professional societies. Increasingly, however, the public demands that physicians not only demonstrate initial competency to practice medicine, but show objective and measureable evidence of life-long learning. In many countries, physicians are being issued time-limited certificates and required to recertify on a regular basis. Recertification entails documenting a certain number of continuing education credits and passing a written examination.

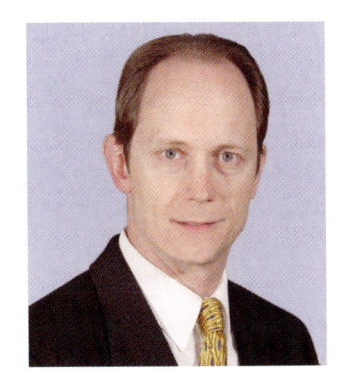

To maintain objectivity and ease of grading, most written qualifying examinations have a multiple-choice question and answer format. The questions can be validated in field-testing and their difficulty can be assessed by the correct response percentage. When used in review format, multiple-choice questions are an excellent way of reinforcing known information and exposing areas of cognitive deficit that require additional study. A problem of the multiple-choice format is that the correct answer is among the distracters, and it is possible to choose the correct answer simply by guessing. If there are n possible answers to a given question, there is a $1/n$ chance that the correct answer can be selected randomly. The odds improve if one or more distracters can be eliminated.

Open-ended questions, on the other hand, require test takers to recall information that has been committed to memory. If such questions are written well, they not only require a recollection of facts, but application of the facts in a problem-solving mode. There are many difficulties in writing questions that have a limited number of possible answers. In fact, the more knowledgeable the test taker, the more often he or she will perform poorly on such an examination because their knowledge makes them aware of the nuances and vagaries of a variety of possible etiologies and courses for any given clinical presentation.

Drs Amar Agarwal, Dimple Prakash and Athiya Agarwal have assembled a collection of patients and clinical scenarios from which they draw relevant evaluation and management questions. This text should be useful for those studying to certify in ophthalmology and those already in practice who are looking for a quick question and answer text to refresh and update their knowledge. The editors are to be congratulated for their effort in producing this text, and for their many other contributions to the field of ophthalmology.

To those who will use this text as a self-study manual, I encourage you to provide feedback to the editors so that they can continue to refine their questions and answers for future editions.

Kevin M Miller MD
Kolokotrones Professor of Clinical Ophthalmology
Jules Stein Eye Institute
David Geffen School of Medicine at UCLA
Los Angeles, California, USA

Foreword to the First Edition

The evaluation techniques have been put to a critical scrutiny for a long time. Clinical assessments apart from being a long and tiring process leave transparency and bias factor a point of discussion. Short and multiple choice question formats have reduced the bias and increased transparency to a great extent in testing the cognitive skills. Objectively Structured Clinical Examination (OSCE) has been visualised as clinical evaluation techniques to eliminate the ambiguity and bias in the clinical examination.

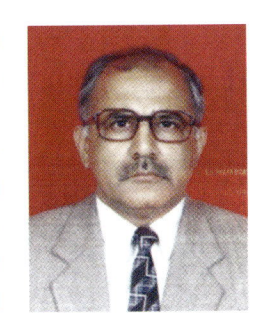

This book is the first attempt to prepare a sample module to introduce OSCE to the students of Ophthalmology. It contains good illustrations along the discrete questions framed to reach with their clear reply. The book has a good learning material as well as clear and critical analysis of the content there in.

I am sure that this book will justify its publication and help to promote OSCE as a friendly induction of a good evaluation technique.

DK Mehta
Director, Guru Nanak Eye Centre
Director, Professor of Ophthalmology
Maulana Azad Medical College
New Delhi, India

Preface to the Second Edition

When we wrote the first edition of the OSCE book, it was the first book published on OSCE. The book helped many students who wanted to sit for their postgraduate exams. Since then we have the annual Kalpavriksha meet in the first week of October every year which is an annual conference for postgraduate training. The word Kalpavriksha means a tree of knowledge. To help students benefit more we decided to bring out the second edition of the OSCE book.

In this edition, we wanted to cover up topics like plastics, microbiology and other interesting topics which are normally covered in the actual OSCE exams. The idea here is basically for you dear readers to understand how the OSCE pattern is and how to succeed in the exam.

We would like to thank all the doctors of Dr Agarwal's Group of Eye Hospitals who helped us prepare this book.

We would also like to thank Shri Jitendar P Vij (Chairman and Managing Director) and the whole team of Jaypee Brothers Medical Publishers (P) Ltd, New Delhi for bringing out such a book.

Amar Agarwal
Dimple Prakash
Athiya Agarwal

Preface to the First Edition

Including OSCE (Objectively Structured Clinical Examination) into the DNB examination is an applaudable decision as it enhances the quality of the examinations and evaluates the performance of the students in a very practical and unbiased manner.

On the other hand, students are not trained for this kind of examination and there is an acute need for more literature on the type of questions asked and appropriate responses. This book seeks to equip the students with a suitable knowledge of the system and to enhance their performance in the examination.

The first of its kind, this book will prove invaluable to all the postgraduate students whether Primary DNB, DO or MS. It will also make interesting reading for examiners.

It is a pleasure to present you this indispensable guide to the OSCE.

Amar Agarwal
DP Prakash
Sunita Agarwal
Athiya Agarwal

Contents

SECTION 1
QUESTION PAPERS 1-25 1

SECTION 2
QUESTION PAPERS 26-50 53

SECTION 3
QUESTION PAPERS 51-75 105

SECTION 4
QUESTION PAPERS 76-100 157

SECTION 5
OBSERVATION STATIONS 209

Section 1

Question papers 1 to 25

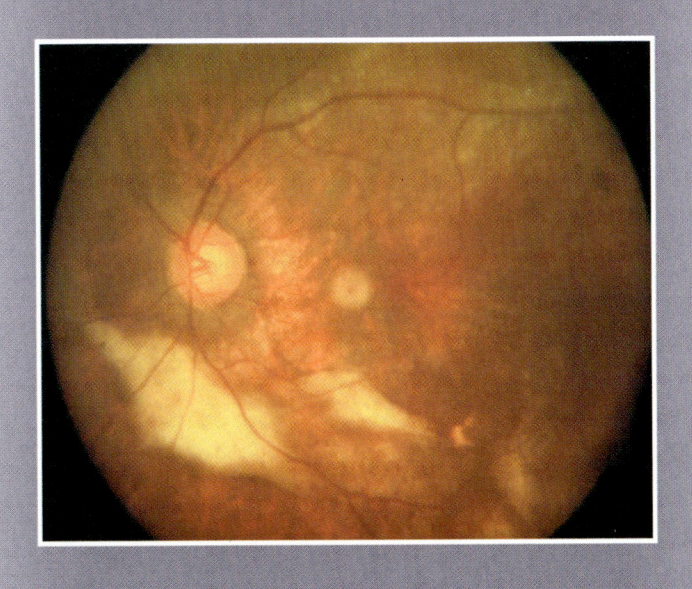

QUESTION 1

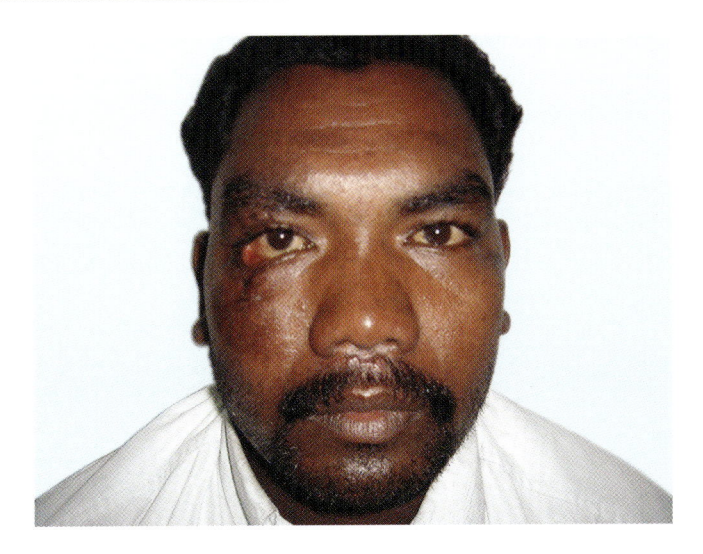

1. What will be the diagnosis of this patient?
2. Mention two complications that this patient will develop if left untreated.
3. In this patient what will be the two surgical procedures of choice?
4. In case of grafting which are the preferred areas of procuring the graft?

ANSWERS

1. This patient has a cicatrical ectropion.
2. Two common complications of untreated ectropions are: Corneal exposure keratopathy and keratinisation of conjunctiva.
3. Two commonly performed surgeries are: For mild cicatrical ectropion – Z or VY plasty and for severe ectropion – split skin grafts of full thickness skin grafts with release of the cicatrix.
4. Grafts are commonly taken from: Posterior auricular, preauricular and supraclavicular areas.

QUESTION 2

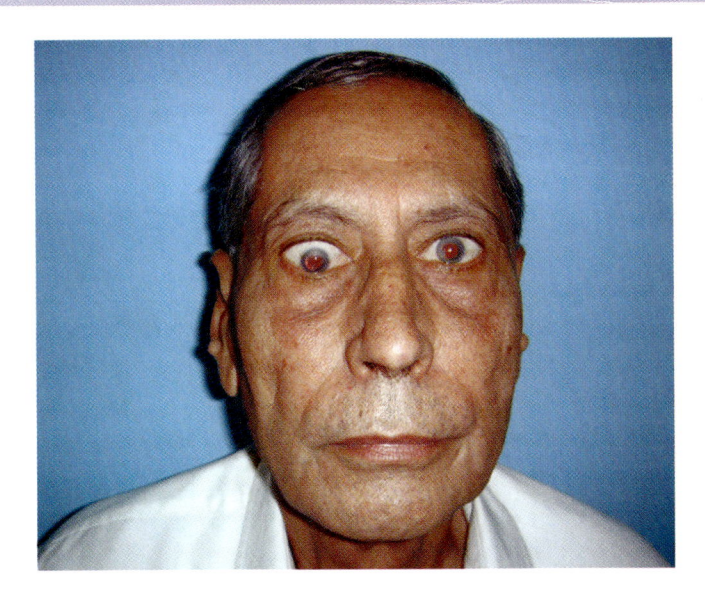

1. Name the lid signs in thyroid eye disease related to the retraction of the eyelid.
2. What percentage of patients with Grave's disease develop thyroid eye disease and what is the risk factor involved?
3. Give the five main clinical manifestation of the disease and state the two stages.
4. What are the causes of visual loss in a patient with thyroid ophthalmopathy?

ANSWERS

1. The three eyelid signs associated with retraction of the lid are: Dalrymple's sign (lid retraction in primary gaze), Kocher sign (staring, frightened look) and von Graefe's sign (slow or restricted descent of the lid on attempted down gaze).
2. 25 to 50% of patients with Graves' diseases develop thyroid eye disease. Smoking is the most important risk factor for a Grave's disease patient to develop thyroid eye disease.
3. The five main clinical characteristics are: Soft tissue involvement, restrictive myopathy, optic neuropathy, and proptosis and lid retraction. The two stages of the disease are: Congestive and fibrotic.
4. The commonest causes of vision loss in thyroid eye disease are corneal exposure keratopathy and optic neuropathy.

QUESTION 3

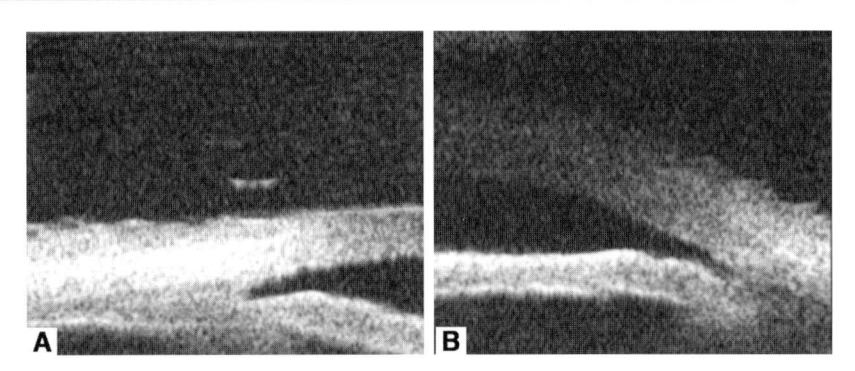

1. What is the imaging shown here?
2. Name the structures visible.
3. What is the other imaging technique by which you can see these structures?
4. What is the advantages and disadvantages of both?

ANSWERS

1. The imaging technique is the UBM : Ultrasound biomicroscopy
2. The structures seen here are the corneoscleral junction, the angle recess, root of the iris and ciliary body with the supraciliary space.
3. Anterior segment OCT is the other imaging technique by which most of these structures can be seen.
4. Advantages of UBM:
   - Study of angle recess and beyond like the ciliary body and the supraciliary space and the suprachoroidal space can be done.
   - Tumors of the iris root, ciliary body with extension can be visualized well.

   Advantages of anterior segment OCT
   - Corneal morphological details seen in detail
   - Easy to learn with shorter learning curve
   - Quick non-contact procedure with greater patient comfort.
   - Anterior chamber cells and reactions seen well
   - Vector measurements possible
   - Serial analysis of disease possible with respect to progress due to ability of data storage.

   Disadvantage of UBM
   - Contact method that requires immersion technique causing patient discomfort and cooperation.
   - Takes a long time to carry out
   - Longer learning curve
   - Vector measurement absent, manual measurement needs to be done
   - Corneal and anterior chamber morphological not seen in detail.

   Disadvantage of anterior segment OCT
   - Iris root and beyond like the ciliary body, supraciliary space and suprachoroidal space not viewed with their details.
   - Lesions and tumors situated beyond the angle recess are not seen well.

QUESTION 4

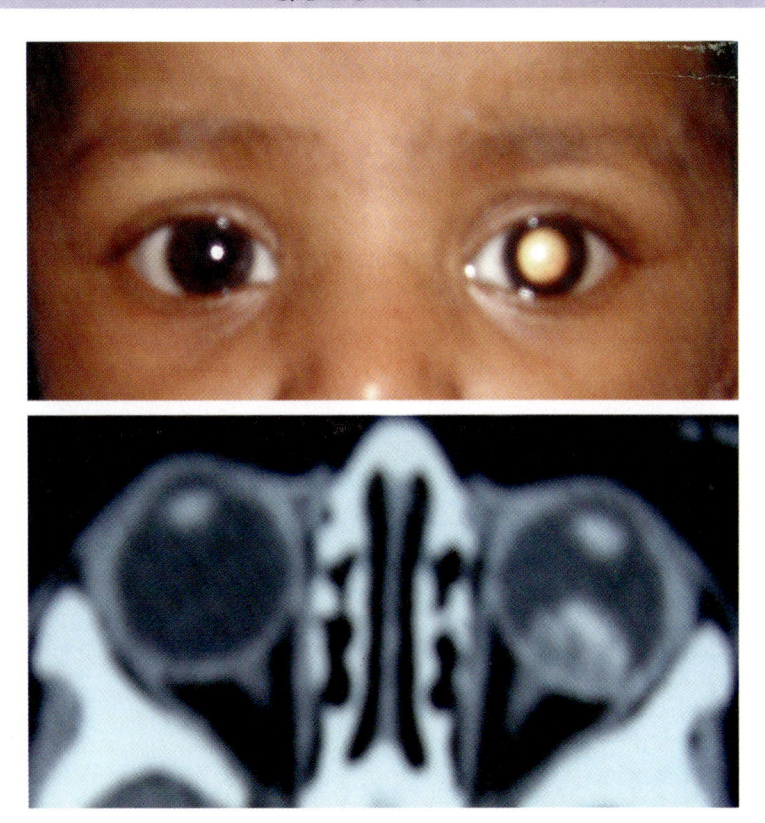

1. What is the most likely diagnosis in this child? What is the other name for the white reflex / leucocoria that is seen here?
2. Give the non-infective causes of pseudoglioma.
3. What is the investigation of choice in this condition? What does the figure show?
4. Which group does this child belong to and why?
5. What will be the vision prognosis of this child? What is the treatment offered to this child?

ANSWERS

1. This child most likely has retinoblastoma. Leucocoria is also called amaurotic cat's eye.
2. Pseudoglioma can be caused by congenital defects like large colobomas, PHPV, Norries disease, retrolental fibroplasias.
3. CT scan is the investigation of choice. The CT scan shows the presence of a intraocular irregular mass extending almost retrolental space with calcification.
4. The child belongs to group 3 on Rees Ellsworth classification. The reason is because the tumour is single, larger than 10 DD and is situated behind the equator.
5. The vival prognosis may be poor in this child due to the close approximity to the optic disc. External beam radiation can be thought of before an enucleation.

QUESTION 5

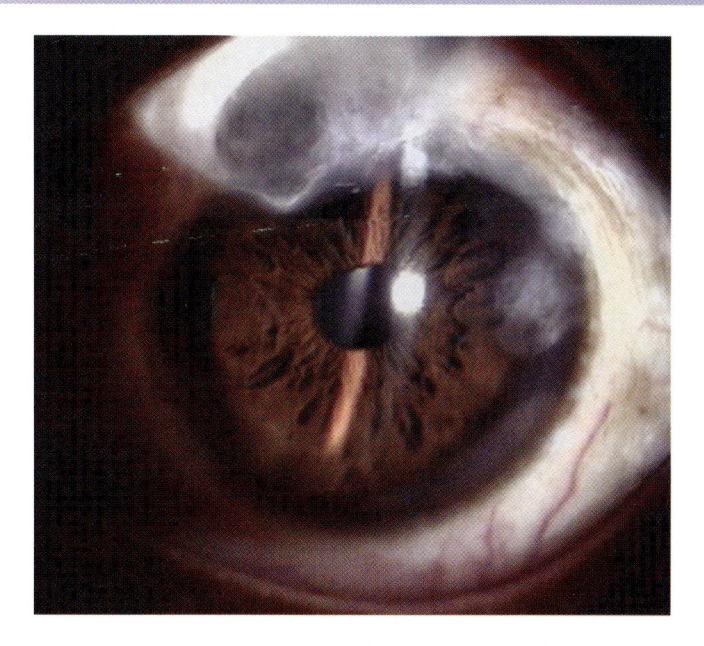

1. Classify and name the surgical procedure that has been performed here. Between which two anatomical spaces is the channel created?
2. What is the type of bleb seen here? Give two reasons.
3. What is the most common cause of failed bleb?
4. What are the non-surgical and non-laser methods of treatment of bleb failure?
5. In what way can laser be used in patients post-trabeculectomy? Name the lens and the lasers that can be used during the procedure.

ANSWERS

1. A partial thickness filtration surgery called trabeculectomy has been performed. The drainage channel is created between the anterior chamber and the sub-tenons space.
2. Overhanging bleb also called over filtering cyst is seen here. It is because
   - It is a localised highly elevated cyst like cavity.
   - There are no engorged surface vessels in the surrounding area.

   Two reasons are – excessive use of antimetabolites during surgery and excessive cautery during surgery.
3. The most common cause of bleb failure is subconjunctival fibrosis.
4. Non-surgical method of bleb failure treatment is digital massage and scleral depression and subconjunctival 5FU injection.
5. The following lasers with the help of Hoskins lens or Zeiss lens can be used:
   - Nd:Yag, for relieving the block at the internal opening of the fistula
   - Argon laser, for laser suture lysis.

QUESTION 6

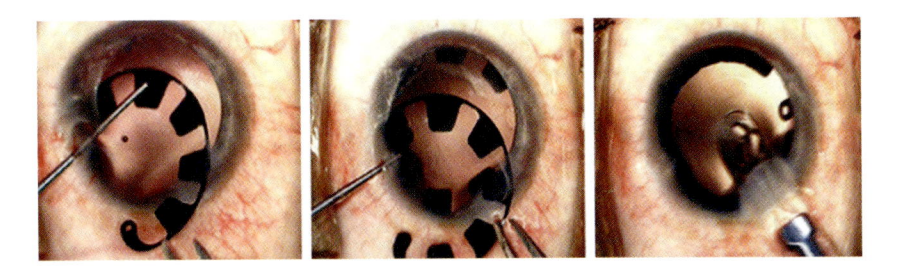

1. What is the name of the implant being put? What are the other types available?
2. Name the clinical condition for which this procedure is being performed. Give its associated lenticular abnormalities.
3. Which other important systemic investigation will you order for this patient? Why?
4. At what age will this patient develop glaucoma and at what percentage?
5. How will the rudimentary stump of iris cause glaucoma?

ANSWERS

1. This implant is called Mocher's implant (Aniridia ring segment).
2. This patient has Anirida, the associated lenticular changes can be: Subluxation of lens, cataract, congenital lens absence, persistent pupillary membrane.
3. Ultrasound of the abdomen should be ordered as Wilms' tumour is commonly associated with Anirida due to the deletion of short arm of chromosome 11.
4. 50 % of patients develop glaucoma and usually found at adolescence and at late childhood.
5. The rudimentary stump will cause glaucoma by closure of the angle with synechiae as a result of contracture of pre-existing fibres between the stump and the angle bridge.

QUESTION 7

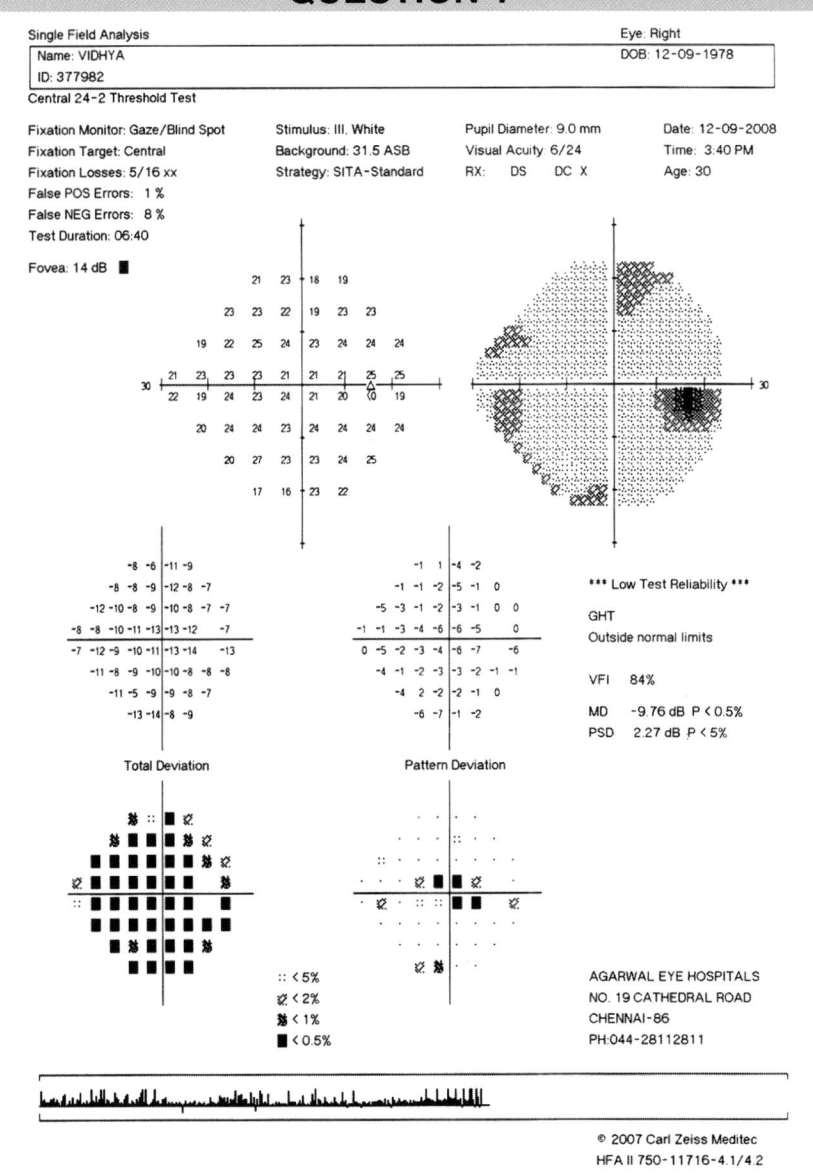

Single Field Analysis
Name: VIDHYA
ID: 377982
Central 24-2 Threshold Test

Eye: Right
DOB: 12-09-1978

Fixation Monitor: Gaze/Blind Spot
Fixation Target: Central
Fixation Losses: 5/16 xx
False POS Errors: 1 %
False NEG Errors: 8 %
Test Duration: 06:40

Stimulus: III, White
Background: 31.5 ASB
Strategy: SITA-Standard

Pupil Diameter: 9.0 mm
Visual Acuity: 6/24
RX: DS   DC X

Date: 12-09-2008
Time: 3:40 PM
Age: 30

Fovea: 14 dB

*** Low Test Reliability ***
GHT
Outside normal limits

VFI 84%
MD -9.76 dB P < 0.5%
PSD 2.27 dB P < 5%

Total Deviation
Pattern Deviation

:: < 5%
< 2%
< 1%
< 0.5%

AGARWAL EYE HOSPITALS
NO. 19 CATHEDRAL ROAD
CHENNAI-86
PH:044-28112811

© 2007 Carl Zeiss Meditec
HFA II 750-11716-4.1/4.2

1. What type of scotoma does this patient have? Name the condition casing this type of visual field defect.
2. Mention the commonest agents causing this clinical condition.
3. What will be the treatment in this patient?
4. Which tests should be done on follow-up of this patient apart from visual fields?
5. What will be the clinical signs on ophthalmoscopy?

ANSWERS

1. This patient has a centroceacal scotoma. The typical condition causing this is toxic optic neuropathy.
2. Commonest causes of toxic optic neuropathy are: Alcohol and smoking.
3. The treatment will be withdrawal of the toxic agent followed by injection of 1000 units of hydroxycobalamin for 10 days along with oral Vit B_{12} and a well balanced diet of proteins.
4. Colour vision, pupillary reactions and near vision test should be done on follow-up visits.
5. Optic disc temporal pallor, mild disc oedema and splinter haemorrhages are the optic disc clinical signs.

QUESTION 8

Appasamy Associates/Gantec Corporation

HOSPITAL INFORMATION:	SUBJECT INFORMATION:
	Name: Test Subject
	Age: 0
	Exam Type: OD
	Diagnosis:
Phone Number:	MRD: 123

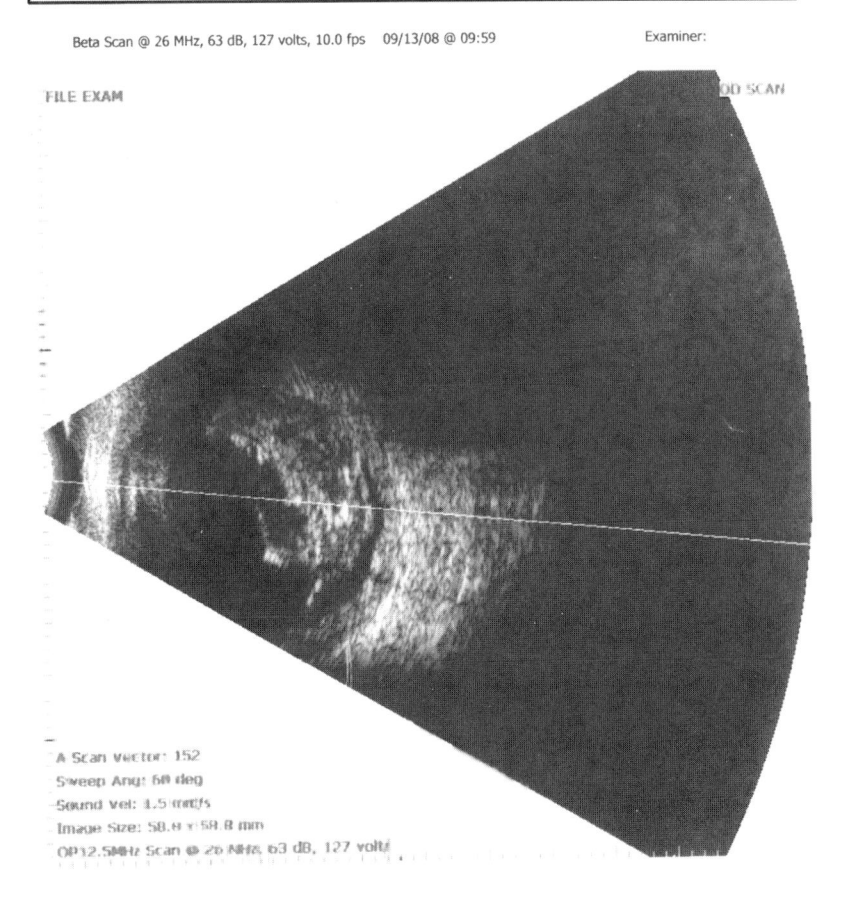

Beta Scan @ 26 MHz, 63 dB, 127 volts, 10.0 fps 09/13/08 @ 09:59   Examiner:

FILE EXAM   OD SCAN

A Scan vector: 152
Sweep Ang: 60 deg
Sound vel: 1.5 mm/s
Image Size: 58.8 x 58.8 mm
OP 12.5MHz Scan @ 26 MHz, 63 dB, 127 volts

1. Differential diagnosis of clinical conditions on this B scan picture.
2. What are the systemic features that can be associated with the above differential diagnosis?
3. What does the A scan picture of this patient show?
4. The retinal blood vessels bleed into which areas of the intraocular cavity?
5. What is the membrane caused by organised blood of vitreous haemorrhage called?

ANSWERS

1. Vitreous haemorrhage, vitreous exudates and asteroid hyalosis are the common differential diagnosis of this B scan picture.
2. The systemic conditions to be thought of in case of vitreous haemorrhage is diabetes mellitus, in case of vitreous exudates systemic causes of uveitis and in case of asteroid hyalosis hypercholesterolemia is to be thought of.
3. The A scan picture in this patient shows moderate spikes.
4. The retinal blood vessels bleed into the intragel, into the subretinal space and into the retinal layers.
5. The organised vitreous haemorrhage blood is called Ochre membrane.

QUESTION 9

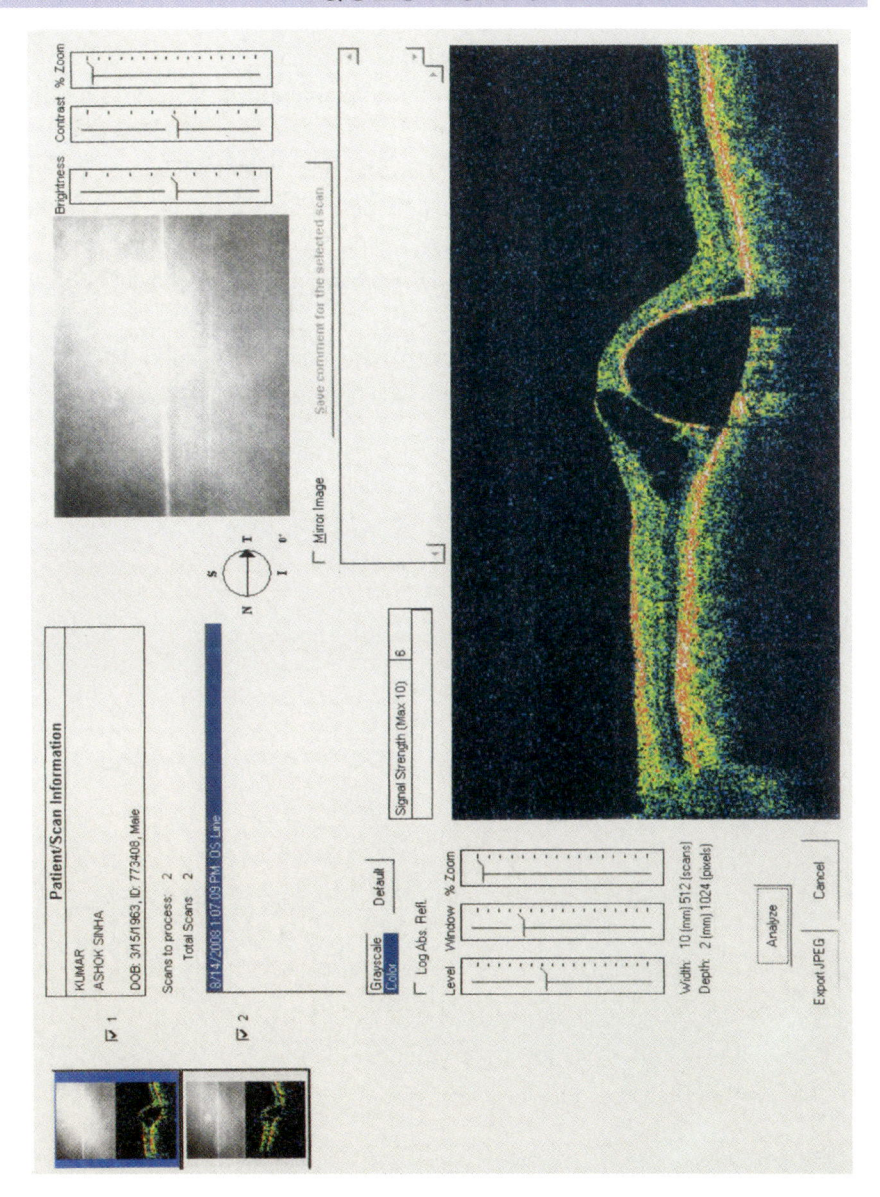

1. Give your diagnosis.
2. Between which layers of the retina is the fluid accumulated?
3. What is the vision threatening complication of this patient? Give your reason.
4. What will be the FFA picture in this patient?
5. What does the red coloured layer signify and why?

ANSWERS

1. This is an OCT showing cystoid macular oedema.
2. The fluid is accumulated between the outer plexiform layer and the inner nuclear layer.
3. This patient can develop a lamellar macular hole which will cause a drop in the vision. The reason of a macular hole developing is the presence of large cystic spaces that are seen on the OCT which will coalesce.
4. The FFA of this patient will show flower pattern appearance due to pooling of the dye causing hyperfluorescence.
5. The red coloured layer is the layer of RPE and choriocapillaries and it is differentiated because of its property of hyper reflectivity.

QUESTION 10

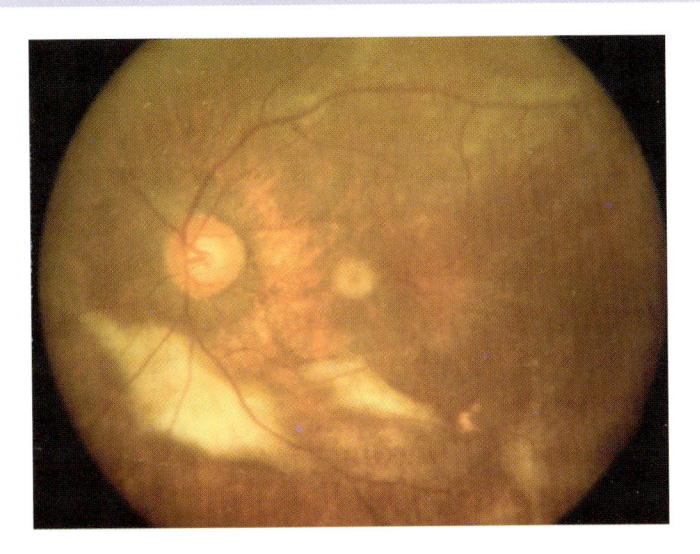

1. Describe this fundus photo and give the diagnosis.
2. Where is the abnormal material deposited and give the reason for it?
3. What are the risk factors of vision loss in this patient?
4. Give two features in case of exudative form of the disease.
5. What will be the FFA picture in this patient?

ANSWERS

1. This fundus photo shows loss of RPE pigmentation and atrophic areas showing the underlying Choroidal vessels. The diagnosis is in the favour of Dry ARMD.
2. The abnormal material is deposited at the level of the Bruch's membrane and it is due to failure of RPE PUMP.
3. The risk factors of vision loss in this patient will be: Large soft drusen, other eye less vision due to ARMD.
4. In exudative form there is RPE detachment and choroidal new vessels.
5. The FFA of this patient will show the presence of hyperfluorescence of choroidal vessels and also window defects.

QUESTION 11

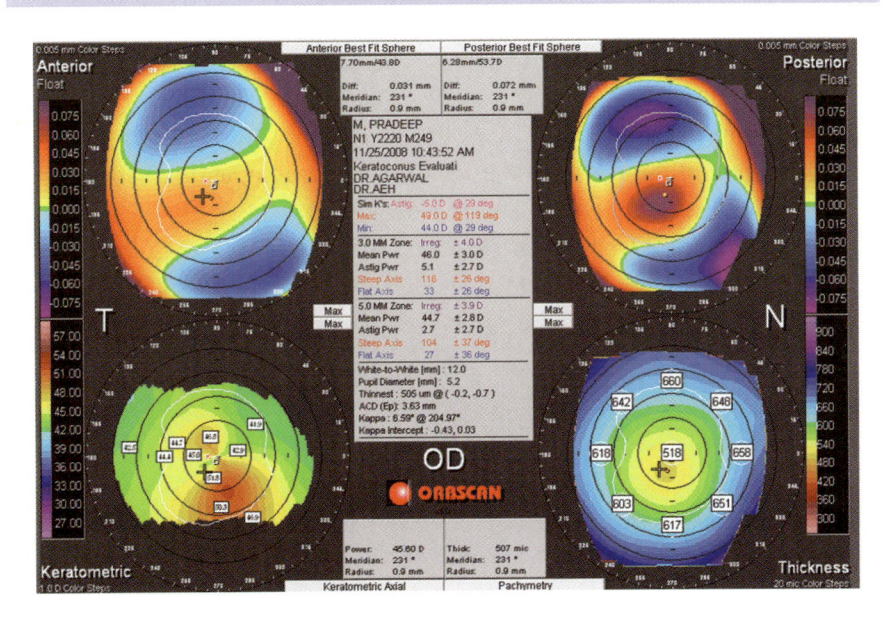

1. What is the astigmatism in the patient?
2. Comment on posterior elevation.
3. Is this patient suitable for lasik surgery? why?
4. What pattern does the astigmatic map shows?
5. What do the numbers inside the circle in the lower right map means?

ANSWERS

1. −5.0 D @ 29 deg.
2. The posterior elevation is seen in left upper map by purple color indicating >0.075 mm elevation.
3. No, because of the ectasia of the anterior and posterior cornea with thinning of the cornea suggestive of keratoconus.
4. Asymmetric Bow Tie with inferior steepening.
5. The numbers inside the circle in the lower left map indicate local corneal pachymetry readings in those areas of the cornea.

QUESTION 12

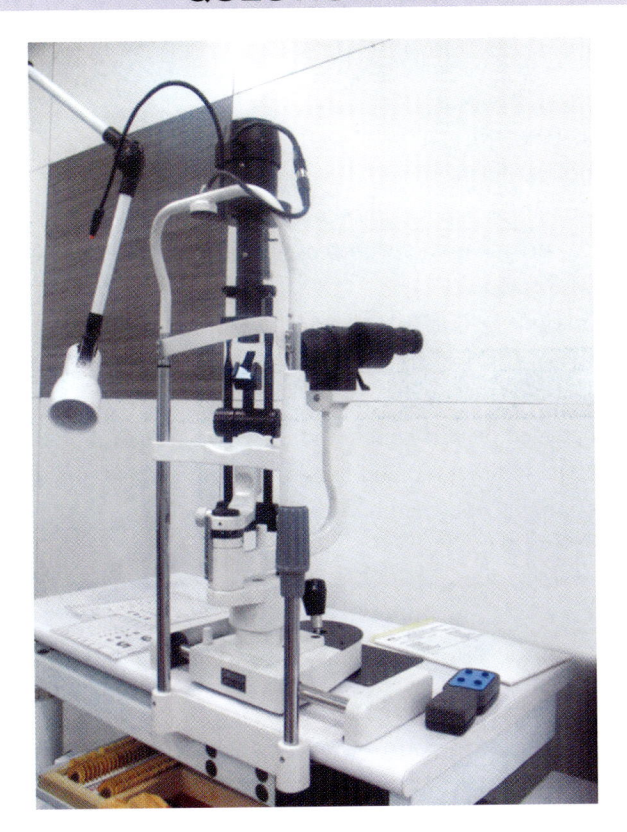

1. Name the parts of this instrument.
2. What are the optical constituents of the microscope and of what power?
3. How many prisms are there in the eye piece and why are they placed there?
4. After whose name is the illumination system named and give the different types of illuminations used?
5. What is the angle between the slit lamp and eye piece on indirect illumination and give four uses of this system?

ANSWERS

1. The three parts of the slit lamp are: Observation system, illumination system and mechanical system.
2. The microscope consists of an objective lens and an eye piece. The objective lens is a set of two planoconvex lenses that add up to a power of 20 diopters. The eyepiece is of 10 and 16 diopters.
3. There are two prisms in the eyepiece; they are there to re-invert the inverted image that is formed.
4. The illumination system is named after Gullstrand and the methods of illumination are: Diffuse, focal, retro, specular, indirect, sclerotic scatter and oscillatory.
5. The angle between the slit lamp and the eyepiece should be between 30 and 45 degrees. The indirect method is used for seeing corneal vacuoles, corneal infiltrates, epithelial cells and microcysts of the cornea.

QUESTION 13

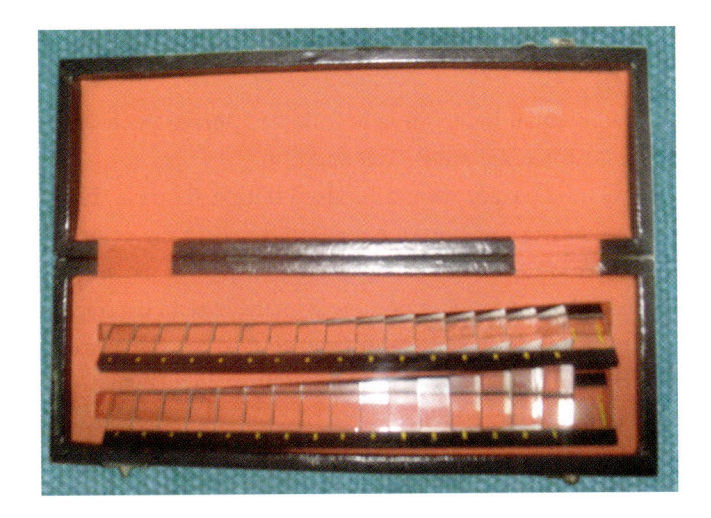

1. Identify this instrument. What is the name of the test done with it?
2. What law of muscle movement does this test follow? What is the distance at which this test can be done?
3. Should an accommodative target be used during this test? Give your reason.
4. How is it placed in front of the eye? What is the end point of the test?
5. What deviation does this test measure?

ANSWERS

1. This is a prism bar. The test is called prism bar cover test or prism bar alternate cover test.
2. Herring's law of equal innervation is followed during the test. The distances at which this test is done are 33 cm and 6 mt.
3. An accommodative target should be used during the test. The reason is so that the accommodation of the patient is controlled during squint measurement and accommodation does not bring about a change in the angle of squint.
4. The prism bar is held in front of one eye with the base in the opposite direction of the squint. The end point during the test is reached when there is no movement of either eye seen or less commonly also when a movement in the opposite direction maybe seen.
5. It measures the total deviation, i.e. manifest and latent deviation.

QUESTION 14

1. What is the name of the test done here? What are the findings?
2. Early glaucomatous changes are seen on which type of visual field testing? Should it be done for this patient?
3. Which stage of glaucoma does this patient belong to? What will be the most likely visual field of this patient?
4. What does the black line indicate? What are the two zones and what should be the normal position or pattern of the black line?
5. What are the other methods of scanning of the optic nerve?

ANSWERS

1. The test done here is the optical coherence tomography. It shows the presence of thinning of almost all the quadrants of the nerve fibre layer and the loss of the double hump pattern.
2. Early visual fields involve testing blue targets on yellow background. It is not recommended in this patient.
3. This patient belongs to late stage of glaucoma. The patient most likely will have a double arcuate scotoma.
4. The black line indicates the patients RNFL distribution. The two zones are the red and green, indicating the area of thinning and the normative thickness of the RNFL respectively. The black line should always be above the red zone with a characteristic double hump pattern.
5. The other methods of scanning in this patient are polarimetry and scanning laser ophthalmoscopy.

QUESTION 15

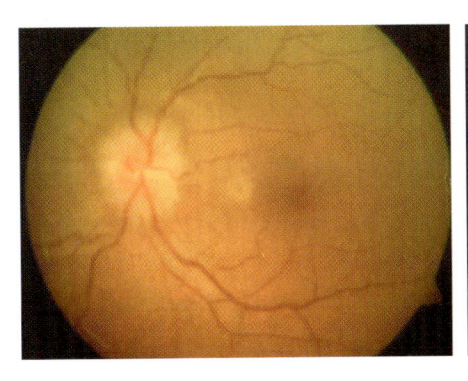

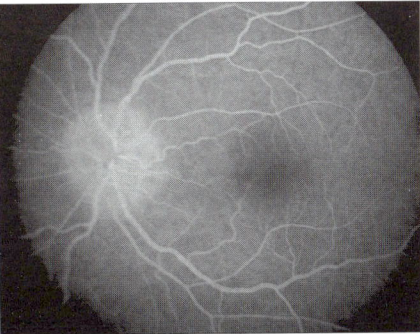

1. Describe the fundus and the FFA pictures.
2. Give your differential diagnosis of this patient.
3. If this was a bilateral condition mention its causes.
4. Mention the ocular causes of this condition of the optic nerve head causing secondary swelling.
5. Mention the conditions causing sudden vision loss in such a patient.
6. If there was optic atrophy in the other eye then what are the conditions called?

ANSWERS

1. This is a fundus picture of the optic nerve head showing blurring of the disc margins, hyperemia of the disc and obliteration of the cup disc ratio. The surrounding area as well as the vessels on the disc appears normal.
   The FFA picture shows hyperfluorescence of the disc.
2. The differential diagnosis of this patient is: Papilloedema, papillitis, AION, hypertensive optic nerve disease and diabetic optic neuritis.
3. Bilateral diseases are seen in raised intracranial tension, hypertension, diabetes, thyroid and cavernous sinus thrombosis.
4. Ocular causes causing secondary disc swelling are:
   - Neuro retinitis and phlebitis
   - Ocular hypotony
   - Ischemic CRVO.
5. Conditions causing of sudden vision loss in this patient are: AION, Papillitis, and ischemic CRVO.
6. Optic atrophy in the other eye are called Foster Kennedy syndrome or psuedo Foster Kennedy syndrome.

QUESTION 16

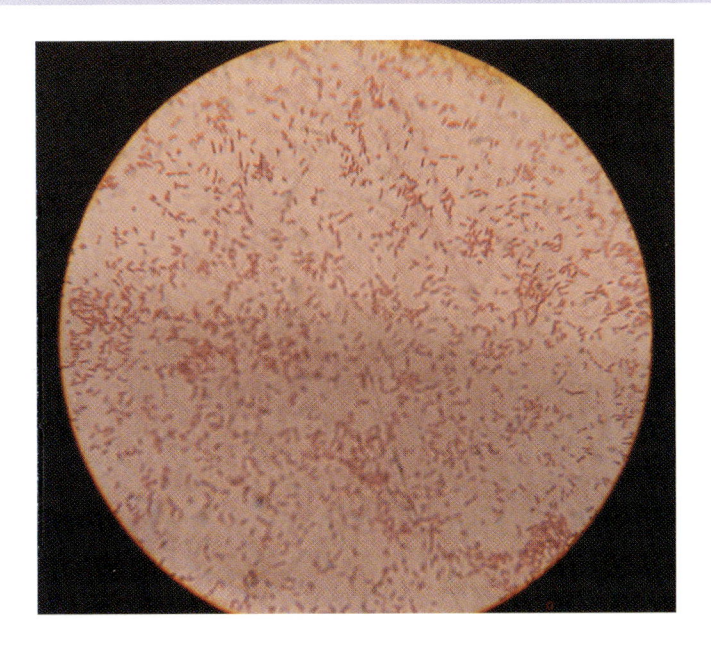

1. Identify the staining and describe the organism. What is the most likely diagnosis?
2. What is the color of hypopyon caused by this organism?
3. Is it motile or non-motile organism?
4. Mention one pigment released by this organism.

ANSWERS

1. The staining used is Gram's staining, the slide shows the presence of pink rod shaped bacilli that are gram-negative, most likely and commonly to be *Pseudomonas*.
2. The color of the hypopyon produced is Green.
3. They are motile organisms.
4. Pyocynine is the pigment released by them.

QUESTION 17

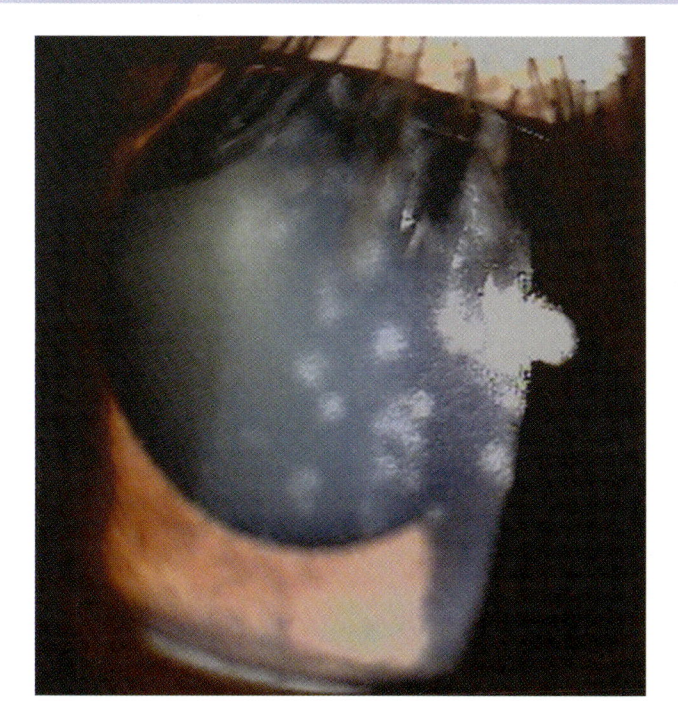

1. Describe the clinical photo and give your likely diagnosis.
2. Mention other aetiologies of similar clinical picture.
3. Which ganglion will lodge the HZ virus? Which are the branches of the trigeminal nerve that will be affected?
4. What is the oral treatment of recurrent herpetic eye diseases, mention dosage and period? What is the treatment of scarred eyes and after how long?
5. Why will a patient get 800 mg of oral Acyclovir five times a day? Give three reasons.
6. Give the role of steroids topical and oral in treatment of viral keratitis.

ANSWERS

1. The clinical photo shows the presence of multiple punctate epithelial and subepithelial lesions involving mostly the anterior layer of the cornea and stroma. The most likely diagnosis is viral keratitis.
2. Other causes of similar clinical picture are:
   - Staphylococci toxin secondary to blepharitis
   - Chemical toxic epitheliopathy
3. The HZ virus is lodged in the Gasserian ganglion. The branches of the trigeminal nerve that are involved are supraorbital, supratrochlear, infratrochlear and nasal.
4. Herpetic recurrent eye disease is treated with oral acyclovir of 400 mg twice a day for six months. Scarred eyes are treated with PTK and PK after a period of one year.
5. 800 mg of Acyclovir are started for the following reasons:
   - Virus shedding period is decreased
   - Healing is accelerated by 50 %
   - Postherpetic neuralgia is decreased.
6. Topical steroids cause reduction in the scarring and are indicated in associated uveitis or scleritis. Oral steroids are indicated in third nerve paralysis, proptosis, optic neuritis and disciform keratitis.

Section 1 37

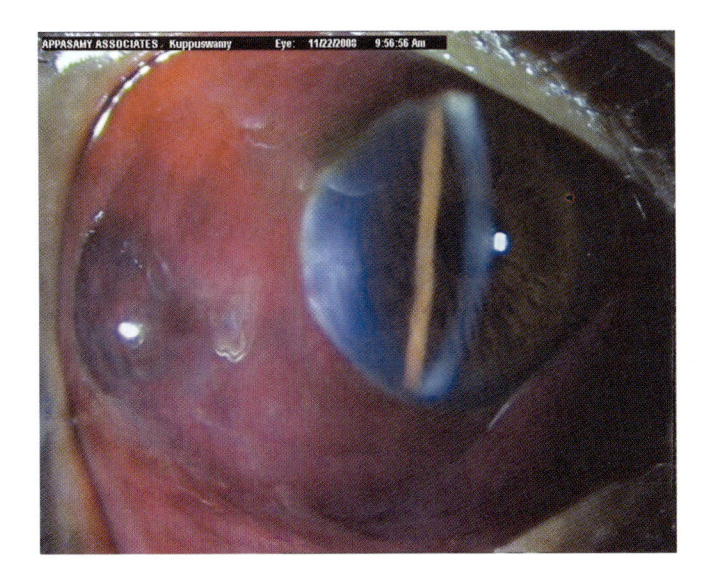

QUESTION 18

1. What is the most likely diagnosis of this clinical picture?
2. If there is iris distortion crescent how will it be differentiated from an iridodialysis?
3. What will be the cause of decreased vision?
4. What is the most suspicious sign seen on the anterior surface of the eye?
5. Describe the diagnostic picture on the B and A scan.

ANSWERS

1. The clinical photo most likely shows an ocular tumour belonging to uveal melanoma with extraocular spread.
2. The iris distortion crescent of a tumour will be differentiated from iridodialysis with the absence of red reflex on transillumination and also absence of H/o of trauma.
3. The cause of decreased vision will be displacement and distortion of lens as well as ciliary muscle malfunction.
4. The anterior surface shows the presence of Sentinel vessels which are the dilated perforating branches of the anterior ciliary arteries.
5. B scan picture shows a classic mushroom shape with A scan showing rapid attenuation of signals and large angle Kappa.

QUESTION 19

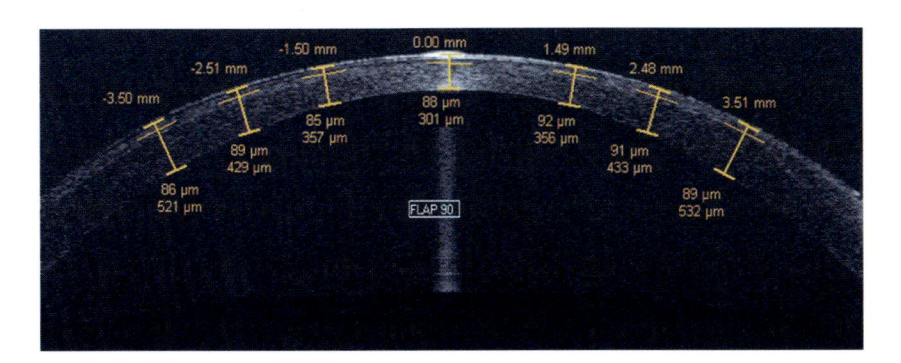

1. Which laser is used in intralase and what is its wavelength?
2. Give 3 etiological factors for diffuse lamellar keratitis.
3. Describe 2 advantages of intralase over microkeratome.
4. Mention 3 patterns of corneal graft edges made by intralase.

ANSWERS

1. Laser used is Nd: YLF, wavelength is 1053 nm.
2. Common causes of DLK are: Meibomitis, bacterial endotoxin, marker ink, microkeratome blade debris, preservatives in drops, interface hemoglobin.
3. The advantages of intralase are: can make thinner flaps, less flap complication, and uniform depth of flaps possible without the meniscus shape.
4. The patterns of corneal grafts that are possible with intralase are: Mushroom pattern, zigzag pattern, top hat.

QUESTION 20

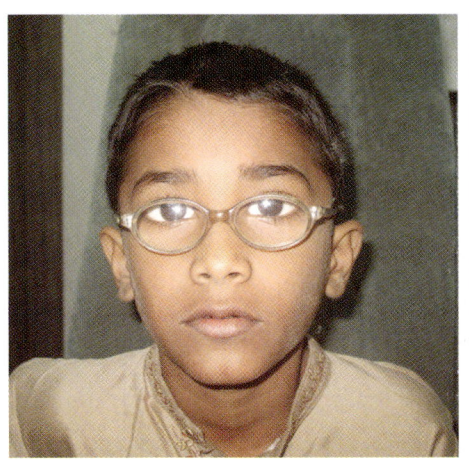

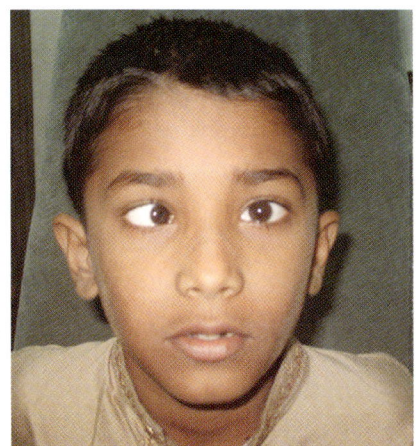

1. What is your complete diagnosis?
2. Define AC/A ratio. How is it measured?
3. State the significance of measuring AC/A ratio in this child.
4. On which examination does the type of surgery to be done depend on, and what are the surgical procedures that can be performed?
5. How much of esotropia should be surgically corrected? What precaution should be taken before surgery?

ANSWERS

1. This child has refractive fully accommodative esotropia.
2. AC/A ratio is defined as the amount of convergence measured in prism per unit diopter change in accommodation. It is measured by the gradient method and the heterophoria method.
3. The significance of AC/A ratio is that it helps to know whether the squint is non-refractive accommodative or refractive accommodative squint. Thus it deals with the management of the child.
4. Examination of squint at distance and at near is important and also the presence of amblyopia should be confirmed. If the deviation is equal for distance and near, then a recession and resection procedure in one eye followed by that of the other eye should be done. If the deviation is greater for near than distance, then bimedial recessions should be done.
5. The residual squint that is not treatable with glasses should be surgically corrected. Amblyopia should be detected and treated before surgery.

Section 1   43

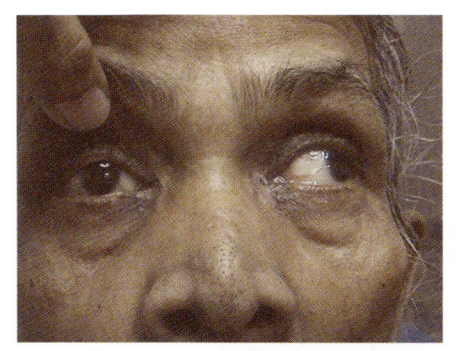

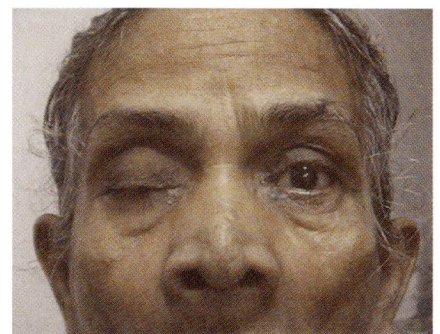

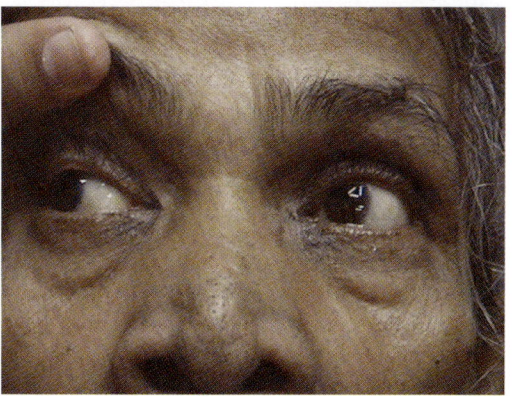

QUESTION 21

1. Give your diagnosis and the clinical findings in the above picture.
2. What are the common causes of the condition?
3. What should be monitored carefully in this patient? State its significance. At what intervals should the follow-up of this patient be placed?
4. What is the most common cause of isolated nontraumatic third nerve palsy with pupillary involvement?
5. What are the signs indicative of cavernous sinus syndrome?

ANSWERS

1. Complete third nerve paralysis. The patient has complete ptosis, exotropia and defective adduction.
2. The common causes of this condition are ischemic, trauma, neoplasm and aneurysm.
3. Pupillary reaction should be carefully monitored. Its significance is that, it is involved in 95% of cases of compressive lesions. It should be monitored every day for the first 5 to 7 days.
4. The commonest cause of isolated third nerve palsy with pupillary involvement is aneurysm at the junction of the posterior communicating artery with the internal carotid artery.
5. Presence of involvement of other cranial nerves namely 4, 5 and 6th along with sympathetic plexus involvement is indicative of cavernous sinus syndrome.

QUESTION 22

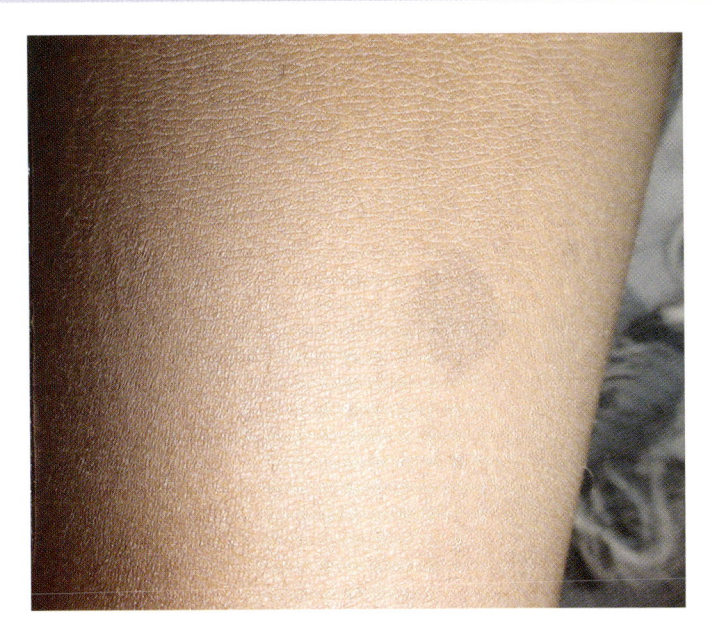

1. What is the likely diagnosis? Which variant of neurofibromatosis are they commonly associated with?
2. Name the two cardinal diagnostics of classic NF1.
3. Give the other skin associations that can be found in neurofibromatosis.
4. Which tumour of the optic nerve is associated with neurofibromatosis?
5. Which clinical picture in patients is commonly associated with glaucoma? Give their percentage.

ANSWERS

1. Café au lait spots and NF type 4 (familial café au lait spots) is the variant of neurofibromatosis that these are associated with.
2. Two cardinal diagnostics of NF are more than 6 café au lait spots and multiple cutaneous neurofibromas.
3. The other skin associations are: Fibrous molluscum, plexiform neurofibromas and axillary freckles.
4. Optic nerve glioma is seen in NF cases.
5. The patients who have *upper lid* and hemifacial hypertrophy are commonly associated with glaucoma and 50% of patients develop glaucoma.

QUESTION 23

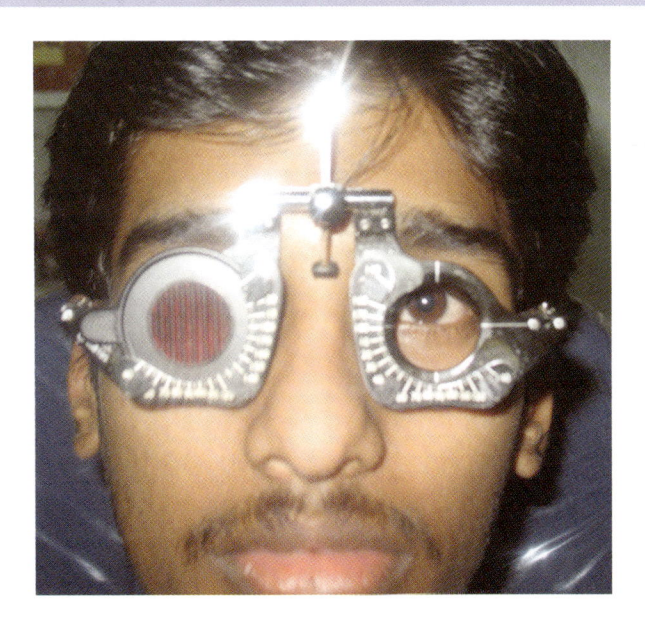

1. At what distance is this test done and it is used to diagnose which type of strabismus?
2. What is the lens made up of?
3. How will you measure the amount of deviation with this test?
4. What is Maddox groove? What is it used for?

ANSWERS

1. This test is done at a distance of 5 to 6 mts. The test diagnoses phorias.
2. The lens is made up of 5 to 6 cut cylinders.
3. The amount of deviation is measured by using the tangent screen or by the strength of prisms placed before the eye to make the dot appear at the centre of the red line.
4. Maddox groove is a red disc with deep grooves on its surface and it is used to measure heterophorias for distance.

QUESTION 24

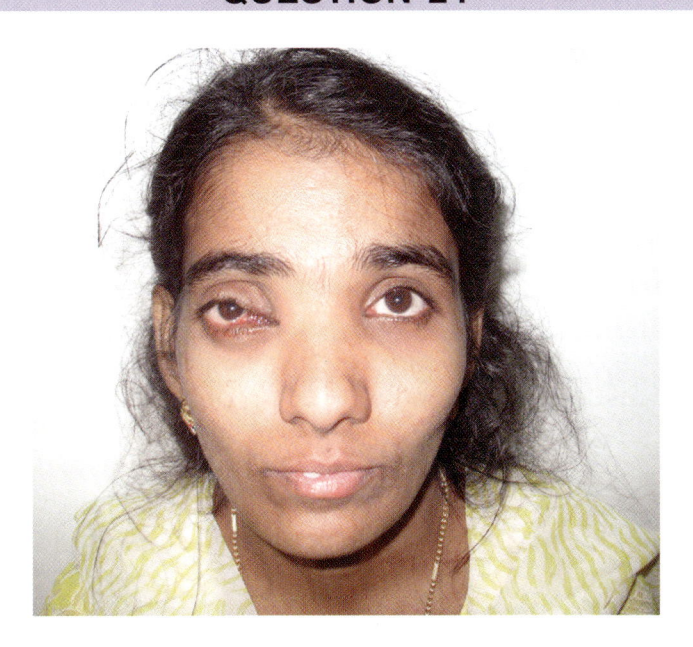

1. Describe the clinical picture.
2. In case of malignancy, give your differential diagnosis.
3. Does this patient have proptosis? If yes, then what type? Give reasons for your answers.
4. What are the types of biopsy possible in this patient?
5. If the surgical excision of the lesion causes a moderate defect then how will it be reconstructed?

ANSWERS

1. This clinical picture shows involvement of the right upper and lower lid with hyperplasia or a mass causing mechanical ptosis and fullness of the upper and lower fornicial spaces. There is also associated proptosis.
2. The following are the differential diagnosis in case of malignancy: sebaceous gland carcinoma and squamous cell carcinoma.
3. Yes the patient has proptosis. It is a non-axial proptosis. The reason for diagnosing proptosis is presence of exotropia with forward displacement of the globe.
4. The two types of biopsy that are commonly done are incisional and excisional. The incisional biopsy is further classified as punch and shave.
5. A moderate sized defect will be reconstructed with a semicircular flap of Tenzel.

QUESTION 25

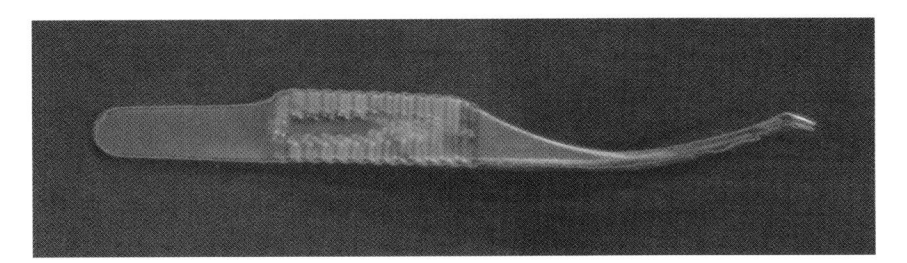

1. Identify the instrument.
2. What are the uses of this instrument?
3. Why is there an angulation present at the tip?
4. What is the significance of the flat area behind the tip?
5. Give another example of similar forceps. Give an example of a less traumatic forceps and the reason for its being less traumatic.

ANSWERS

1. The instrument is Colibri forceps.
2. The uses of the instrument are: Holding tissue like corneal and scleral, *tying the sutures* and fixing the ocular surface tissue while doing surgery.
3. The angulation is present at the tip so as to facilitate easy manipulation of the tissue.
4. The flat area behind the tip is to facilitate easy tying of sutures.
5. A similar forceps is Lims forceps. A less traumatic forceps is Pierce Hoskins; the reason for it being less traumatic is that its two ends appose each other like cups.

Section 2

Question papers 26 to 50

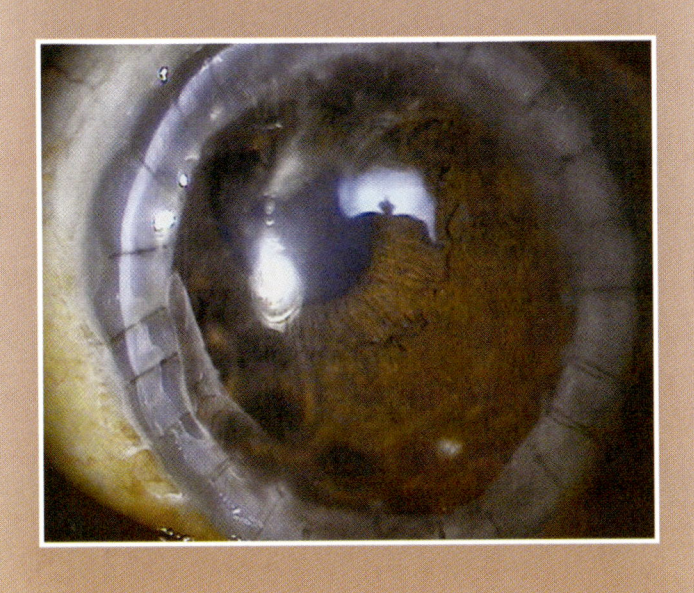

ENTROPION

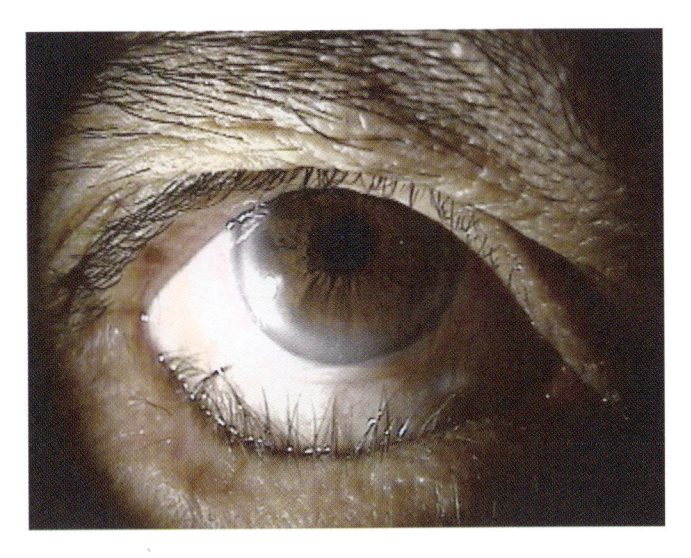

QUESTION 26

1. What does this patient have? Give the three pathogenesis of this condition.
2. Name the two commonly performed surgical procedures in this patient.
3. State the classification of this clinical entity.
4. What is the differential diagnosis if this condition was congenital? How will you differentiate it clinically?

ANSWERS

1. The patient has senile entropion. Three pathogenesis are as follows:
   – Horizontal lid laxity
   – Vertical lid instability
   – Over-riding of preseptal orbicularis over pretarsal orbicularis.
2. Two common surgical corrections will be: Bick procedure modified by Reeh and Jones, Reeh and Wobig procedure.
3. Entropions are classified as follows: involutional, cicatrical, spastic and congenital.
4. Congenital entropions are differentiated from epiblepharon; this is done by pulling the extra-fold of skin away from the lower lid that allows the normal position of the lid margin to become visible in case of an epiblephanon.

QUESTION 27

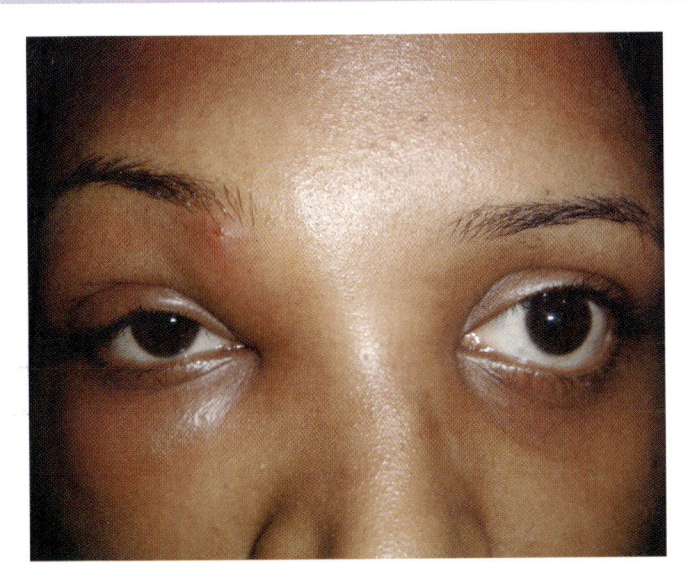

1. What clinical signs will differentiate this condition from orbital cellulitis?
2. Mention the commonest cause of this condition and in what age group is this seen?
3. What is the commonest causative organism in children and in adults in case of orbital cellulitis?
4. What should be monitored carefully at frequent intervals and how?
5. Give the indications of surgical drainage and the radiological investigation of choice.

ANSWERS

1. Tender lid swelling without proptosis is characteristic of preseptal cellulitis. Orbital cellulitis will have proptosis, limitation of ocular movements and involvement of pupillary reactions, all of which are absent in preseptal cellulitis.
2. Preseptal cellulitis is most commonly secondary to acute hordeolum and it is frequently seen in children.
3. The organism most commonly seen in children is *Haemophilus influenzae* and in adults it is *Streptococcus pneumoniae*.
4. Optic nerve function should be monitored frequently at 4 day intervals by observing the pupillary reactions, colour vision and visual acuity.
5. CT scan of the sinuses and the orbit with brain should be done. The indications of surgical drainage are: decreasing vision, nonresolving abscess and subperiosteal abscess formation.

QUESTION 28

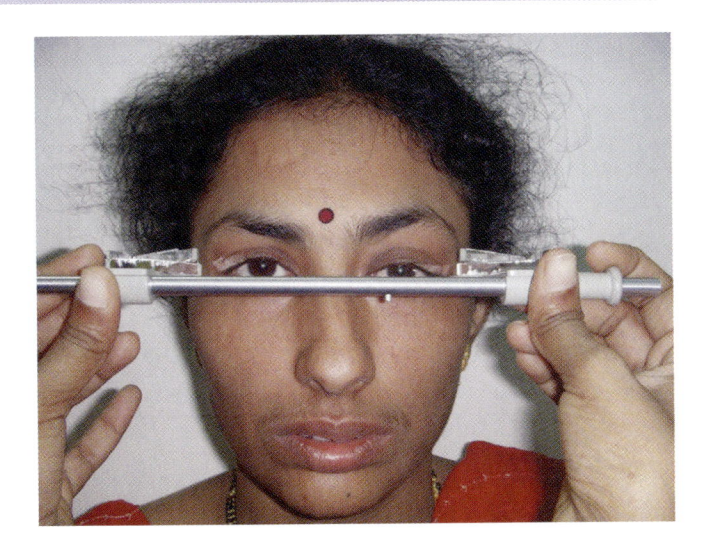

1. What are the other instruments or methods of doing the above test?
2. Is the test shown above is done in right way? If not give two important points while taking the measurements.
3. Mention commonest cause of bilateral proptosis in adult and in a child.
4. The distance between which two anatomical landmarks is measured while doing exophthalmometry.

ANSWERS

1. The other methods of exophthalmometry are the Leude's scale and transparent ruler.
2. No this test is not being done the right way. Two important points to be kept in mind while doing the test are:
   - The examiner has to place the fifth finger at the external auditory meatus for stabilizing the instrument and the examiner should be at the same level as that of the patient; preferably both should be in sitting posture.
3. Commonest cause of bilateral proptosis in an adult is thyroid ophthalmopathy and that in a child is metastatic malignancy like leukemia, neuroblastoma.
4. The distance between the lateral orbital rim and the anterior corneal surface is measured while doing exophthalmometry. The corneal reflex that is seen in the minor of the exophthalmometry is then taken as the reading.

QUESTION 29

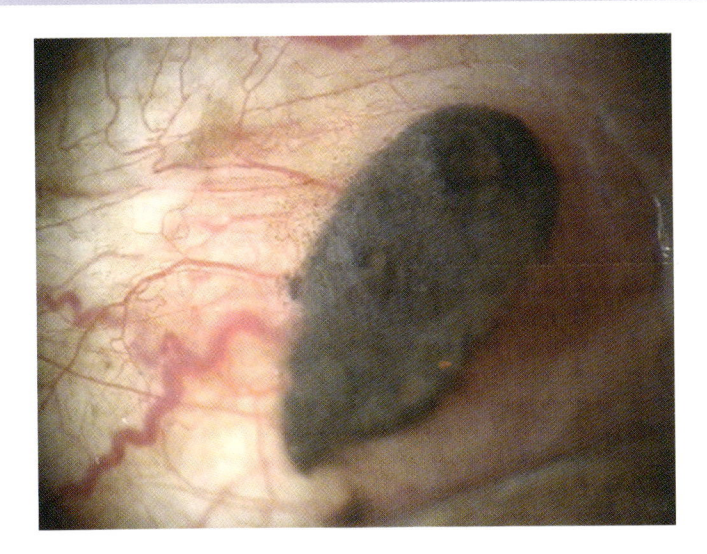

1. What is your diagnosis? What are the three forms?
2. What is this site of the lesion? What are the other sites where it can be present?
3. Can this lesion be multifocal? What are the ways of its presentation? What is the percentage of nonpigmented lesions?
4. When should a lesion situated near the limbus be suspected to be a malignant melanoma?
5. Does this lesion change its colour and size, if so, then normally at what age?

ANSWERS

1. The clinical picture shows a conjunctival nevus. The three forms are intraepithelial, subepithelial and compound.
2. This lesion is situated at the juxta limbal area which is the most common site. The other sites are plica, caruncle and eyelid margin.
3. Conjunctival naevi are never multifocal. They are focal or diffuse. thirty percent of the lesions are nonpigmented.
4. When the juxta limbal lesion encroaches the peripheral cornea a malignant melanoma should be suspected.
5. The lesion is likely to increase in its pigmentation and size at the time of puberty.

QUESTION 30

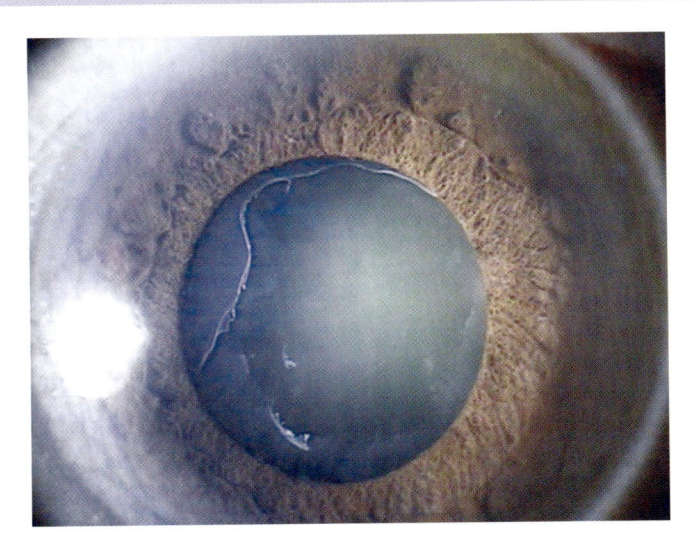

1. What is your diagnosis? Give positive clinical characteristics of the picture?
2. What structure is responsible for the central clear zone and what changes will be seen on that structure?
3. What line is seen on gonioscopy, describe it?
4. Which is the treatment of choice in this condition?
5. What precaution should be taken during cataract surgery in such patients, why and which instrument can be used intraoperatively under such conditions?

ANSWERS

1. This is a clinical picture of Pseudoexfoliation syndrome. The pupillary margin shows deposition of white fibrillary material and the anterior lens capsule shows ring like or wreath pattern deposits of white exudates.
2. The movement of the pupillary margin of the iris on the anterior lens surface produces a central clear zone. Due to constant rubbing of the posterior iris surface on the lens capsule there are transillumination defects that are seen on the iris.
3. The line seen on gonioscopy is called Sampaolesi's line and it is a pigmented line seen anterior to the Schwalbe's line.
4. These patients respond well to ALT.
5. Precaution while cataract surgery should be taken to avoid damage to the zonules of the lens by doing a gentle, central and smaller anterior capsulotomy as the zonules are weak in this condition. The instrument used intraoperatively is called capsular tension rings (CTR).

QUESTION 31

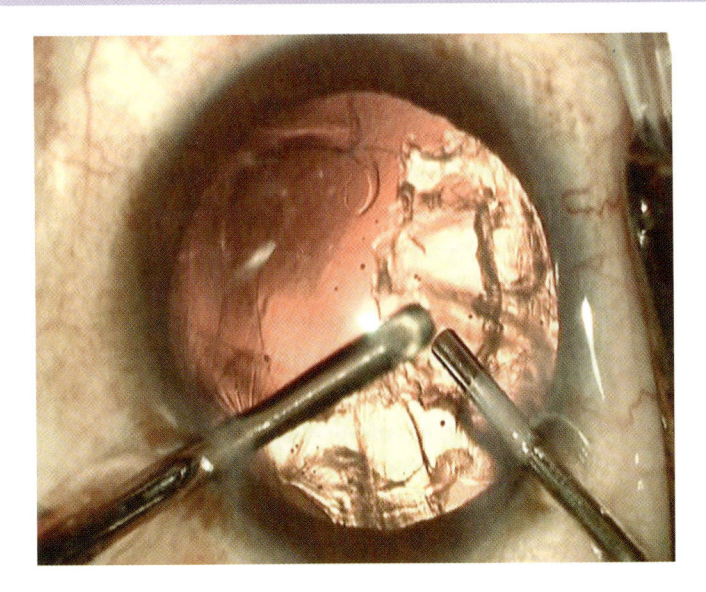

1. What is the surgery being done and which step of surgery is being performed?
2. Which two purposes does the aspiration probe serve?
3. Name the three types of phacomachines.
4. What is the recommended height of the bottle in phacoemulsification and in ECCE and vitrectomy?
5. What is the amount of fluid entering the eye dependent upon and what is the pressure inside the eye dependent upon?
6. What are the advantages of bimanual aspiration?

ANSWERS

1. Phakonit, Irrigation and Aspiration step.
2. The aspiration probe serves two purposes: production of a vacuum and production of suction forces.
3. The three types of phacomachines are peristaltic system, diaphragmatic system and venturi system.
4. The recommended bottle height in phacoemulsification is 65 cm and in case of ECCE is 50 cm and in vitrectomy is 40 cm.
5. The fluid entering the eye depends upon the gravity and the pressure inside the eye. The pressure inside the eye is dependent upon the height of the bottle and the size of the irrigation port.
6. The bimanual aspiration has the following advantages:
   - It causes less astigmatism due to small openings.
   - Allows better manoeuvrability
   - Easy removal of subincisional cortex.

QUESTION 32

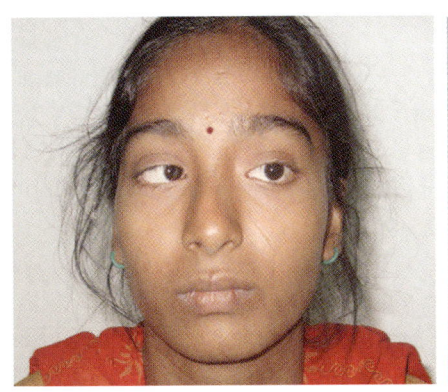

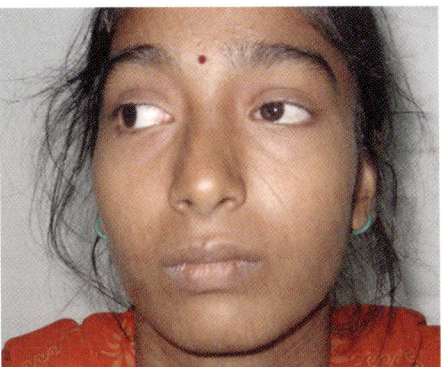

1. What is your diagnosis?
2. Name two syndromes associated with this? Also state the congenital defects that the child can have.
3. What phenomenon is associated with this condition? What is it's treatment?
4. What is the surgical treatment of choice in type 1 and type 2?
5. What is the pathophysiology in this syndrome and why is the resection of lateral rectus contraindicated?

ANSWERS

1. Duane's retraction syndrome type 1.
2. Two syndromes associated with this are: Goldenhar and Wildervanck syndrome. The child can have a hearing or a speech disorder as well.
3. The phenomenon commonly seen is the leash phenomenon and a severe leash is treated with Y splitting of the lateral rectus muscle with posterior fixation sutures of the lateral rectus muscle.
4. Type 1 with an esotropia in primary gaze is treated with medial rectus recession and type 2 with an exotropia is treated with lateral rectus recession.
5. The pathophysiology is the absence of innervation of the lateral rectus by the sixth nerve and abnormal innervation of the lateral rectus by fibres of third nerve. Resection of the lateral rectus should be avoided as it worsens the retraction.

QUESTION 33

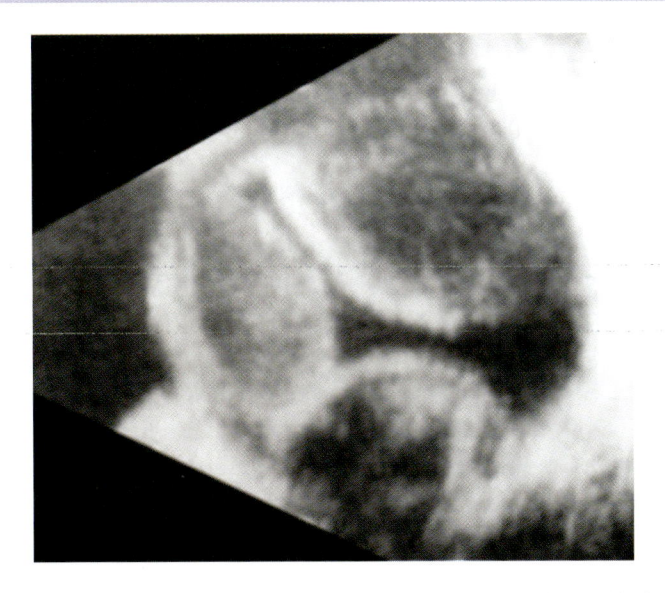

1. Give your diagnosis and what is this presentation typically called.
2. Give three commonest causes of this condition.
3. Which is the intraocular surgery commonly causing this condition and what is the reason?
4. What be the anterior chamber in this patient and what will the pupil of this patient show?
5. Will there be an increase in the IOP in such cases? What is the treatment in long standing cases?

ANSWERS

1. This is an ultrasound (B scan) showing choroidal detachments. They're also called kissing choroidal.
2. Three commonest causes of this condition are; postoperative, tumours and trauma.
3. The commonest intraocular surgery causing choroidal detachment is trabeculectomy with an excessive filtration bleb. The reason is increased vasodilatation that causes exudation of fluid into the outer choroidal lamellae.
4. The anterior chamber in these patients is shallow and the pupil shows a dark mass by oblique illumination.
5. Increased IOP seen in long standing cases of shallow AC is due to iris contact with the peripheral cornea causing synechiae angle closure. The treatment in long standing cases is drainage of the subchoroidal fluid and formation of the anterior chamber.

QUESTION 34

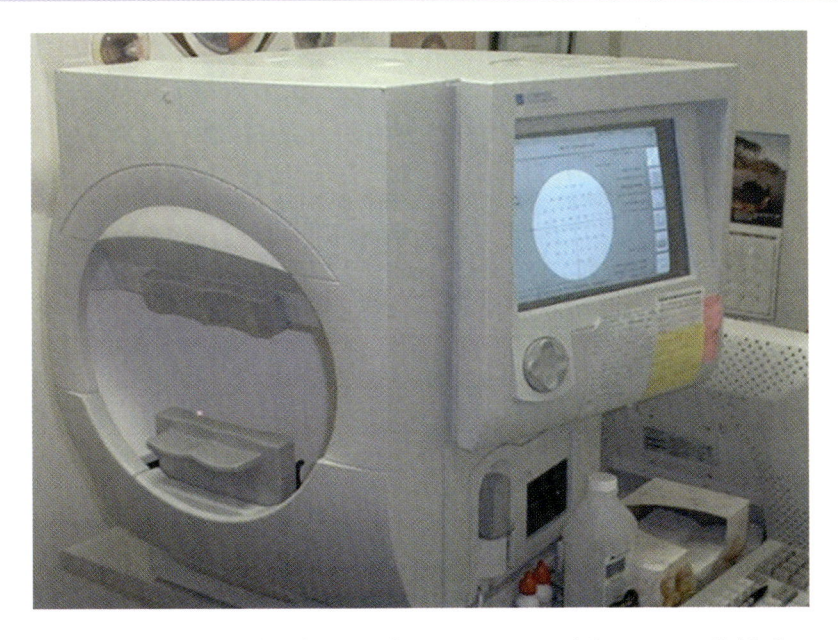

1. Name this instrument? What are the two commercial types available?
2. What are the isopters tested in Goldmann perimetry?
3. Which isopters should be tested with care for early glaucomatous changes?
4. Octopus 32 and Humphrey 30–2 test how many locations?
5. How are the spots in 30–2 and 32 programmes placed and how does this differ from 31 or 30-1 programmes?

ANSWERS

1. This is a computerised automated static perimetry instrument. The two types are Octopus and Humphrey.
2. In Goldmann perimetry the isopters tested are temporal 25 degrees and 15 degrees above and below.
3. Early glaucomatous changes occur in the 5, 10 and 15 degree isopters.
4. The octopus 32 and Humphrey 30-2 test 76 locations in the central 30 degrees of visual field
5. In 30-2 and 32 programmes the spots are arranged in a grid pattern that consists of separation of 6 degrees from each other and 3 degrees on either side of the midline and this differs from the 31 and 30-1 programmes as the spots in them are directly placed on the midline.

QUESTION 35

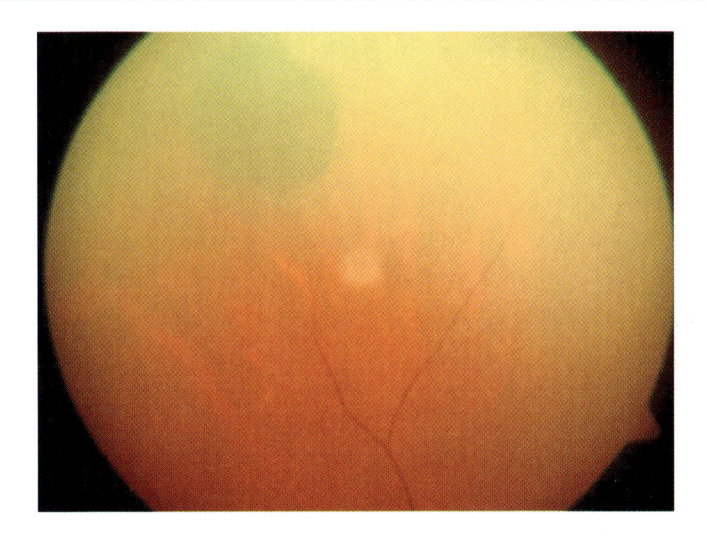

1. What is your 2 differential diagnosis?
2. What are the signs of suspicion in this lesion with respect to size, thickness and surface?
3. What will be the FFA finding in this patient? Which feature on FFA is a suspicious of malignancy?
4. What will be the ICG and the ultrasound picture of this patient?
5. When is the early Biopsy indicated and why?

ANSWERS

1. The differential diagnosis of the patient is Choroidal nevus or Choroidal melanoma.
2. The signs of suspicion are: size more than 5 mm, thickness more than 1 mm, surface lipofuscin and absent drusen.
3. The FFA will show hypofluorescence of the lesion with hyperfluorescence of the drusen. Multiple areas of hyperfluorescence with pinpoint appearance are suspicious of small melanomas.
4. The ICG will show hypofluorescence and U/S will show elevation with high internal reflectivity.
5. Early biopsy is indicated in all atypical as well as suspicious lesions because of early and severe systemic spread that is associated with melanomas by the time they are detected.

QUESTION 36

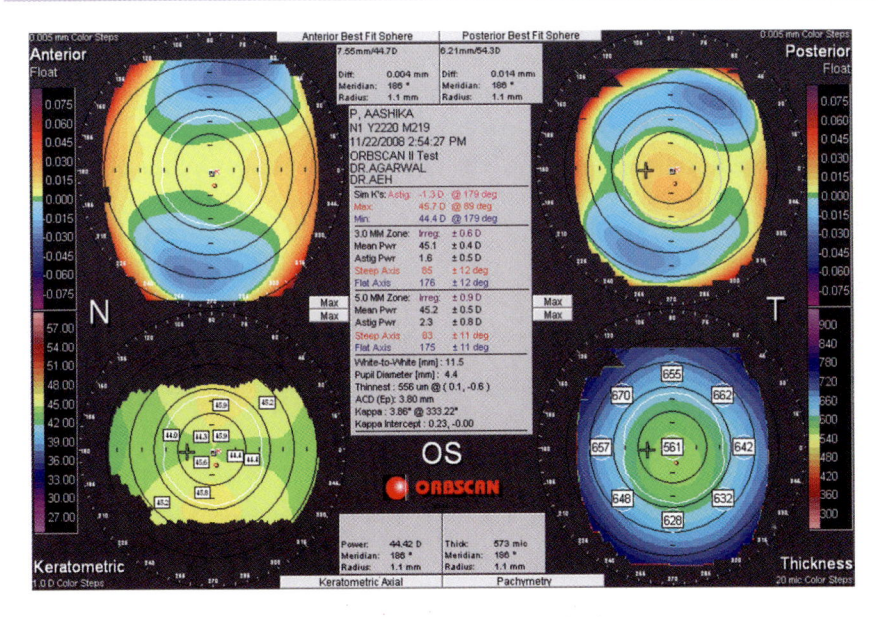

1. What are the 4 indications for corneal topography?
2. What does the upper right and left map indicate?
3. What is the elevation of the anterior best fit sphere?
4. What is the minimum corneal thickness in the patient?

ANSWERS

1. Screening of patient for LASIK, evaluation of keratoconus, IOL power calculation using K value, contact lens fitting (it allows peripheral corneal topographic evaluation).
2. Upper right indicates anterior best fit sphere, upper left indicates posterior best fit sphere.
3. 0.004 mm.
4. 556 µm.

QUESTION 37

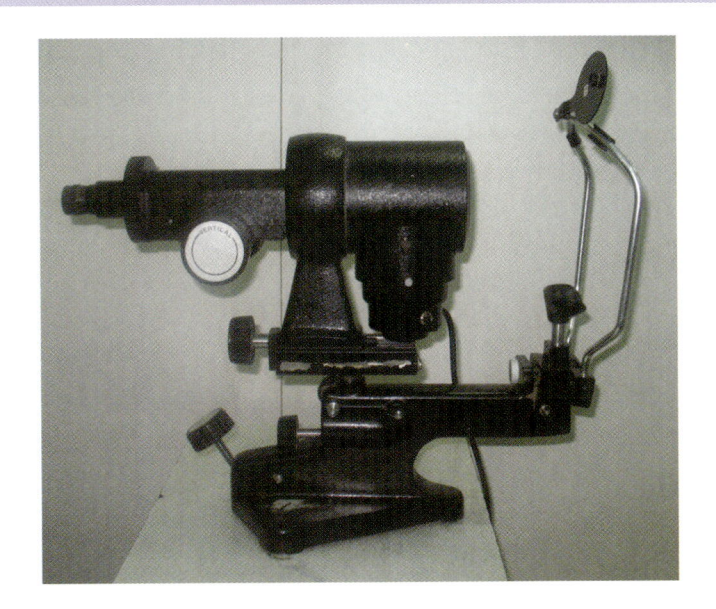

1. How is the corneal optical zone measured?
2. What is the relation between the curvature of the cornea and the image size?
3. What are the three principles of keratometry with their respective types?
4. What is the range keratometry reading that tonometers take? Which image is observed?
5. How are keratometer calculations calibrated?

ANSWERS

1. The optical zone is measured with a fixed chord length of 2-3 mm.
2. The greater the curvature of the cornea, lesser is the image size. So the two are inversely proportional.
3. The three principles with types are as follows:
   - Doubling the image – Helmholtz keratometer.
   - Constant object, variable image – Bausch and Lomb keratometer.
   - Constant image variable object – Javal Schiotz tonometer.
4. The range of keratometry possible is 36 to 52 diopters. The first Purkinje image is observed.
5. Keratometer calculations are calibrated on the refractive index of the corneal that is multiplied by 1.337.

QUESTION 38

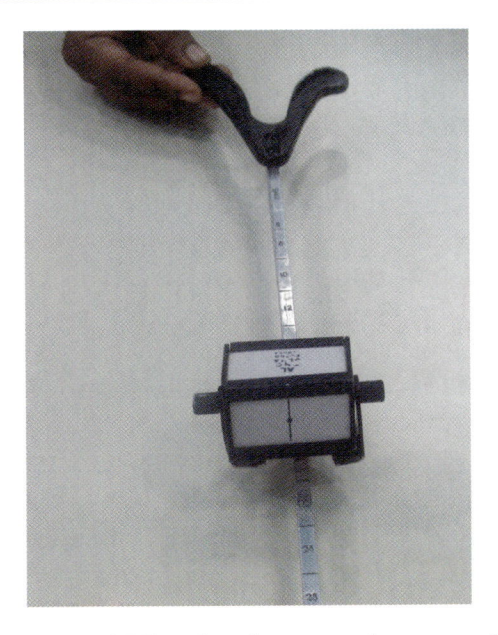

1. What is this instrument? What does it commonly measure?
2. Mention another instrument that can be also be used.
3. What are the two ways that the near points can be measured? State the differences between the two.
4. Give the normal values of NPC? What does blur point indicate?
5. Name three commonly used exercises to treat convergence insufficiency.

ANSWERS

1. This is the RAF ruler, and it is used to test the convergence and accommodation of the patient.
2. Prince ruler can also be used to teat the convergence and accommodation distance
3. The two methods are: objective and subjective. The subjective method is when the patient complains of a blurring while measuring accommodation and doubling while measuring convergence. The objective method is when one eye moves outwards or there is loss of fixation in one eye when the test object is being moved towards the nose.
4. The NPC should be at 8 to 10 cm. Blur point indicates the limit of accommodation, within which clear image can be formed inspite of increased convergence.
5. Convergence insufficiency can be treated with pencil pushups, cat card exercises and SHOT: simple home orthoptics treatment scale.

QUESTION 39

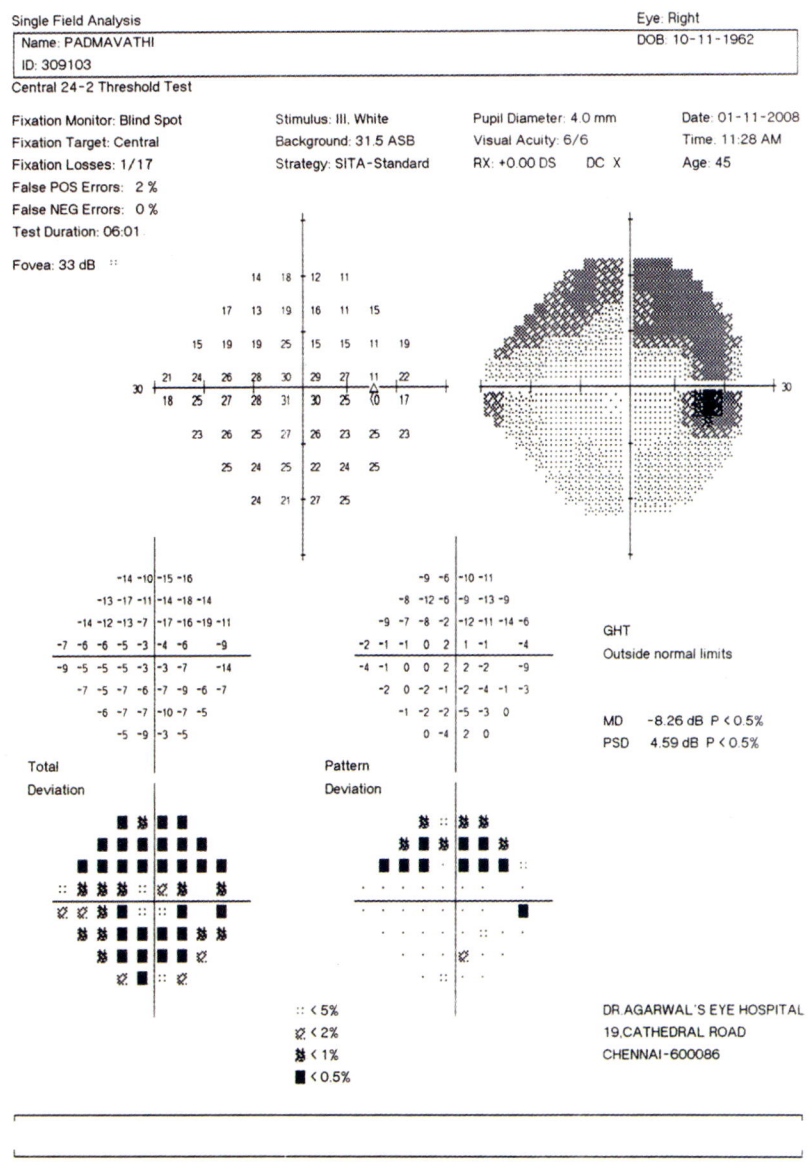

1. Interpret this visual field.
2. Is this field reliable? Give your reasons.
3. What is the difference between short and long-term fluctuation?
4. What are the nonglaucomatous causes of arcuate defects?
5. What is the STATPAC programme?

ANSWERS

1. This is a visual field done using a computerised automated perimeter of Humphrey type, using the SITA standard technique. It shows the presence of an arcuate scotoma in the Bjerrum's area that is continuous with the blind spot, suggestive of glaucomatous visual field defect.
2. Yes the field is reliable. The reliability indices are: false positives and negatives, both of these are lower than 20%, fixation losses are also lower than 20%
3. Short-term fluctuation is tested during the same test. Each of the 10 points are tested twice in the same test. When the points are tested between two separate visual fields at different times then the fluctuation is called long-term.
4. Other causes of visual field defects (nonglaucomatous) are: optic nerve drusen, optic nerve compression, ischemia of the optic nerve and optic neuritis.
5. STATPAC is a programme of the Humphrey system that compares the deviation of the points from the normal along with age matched population, it provides a graphic printout.

QUESTION 40

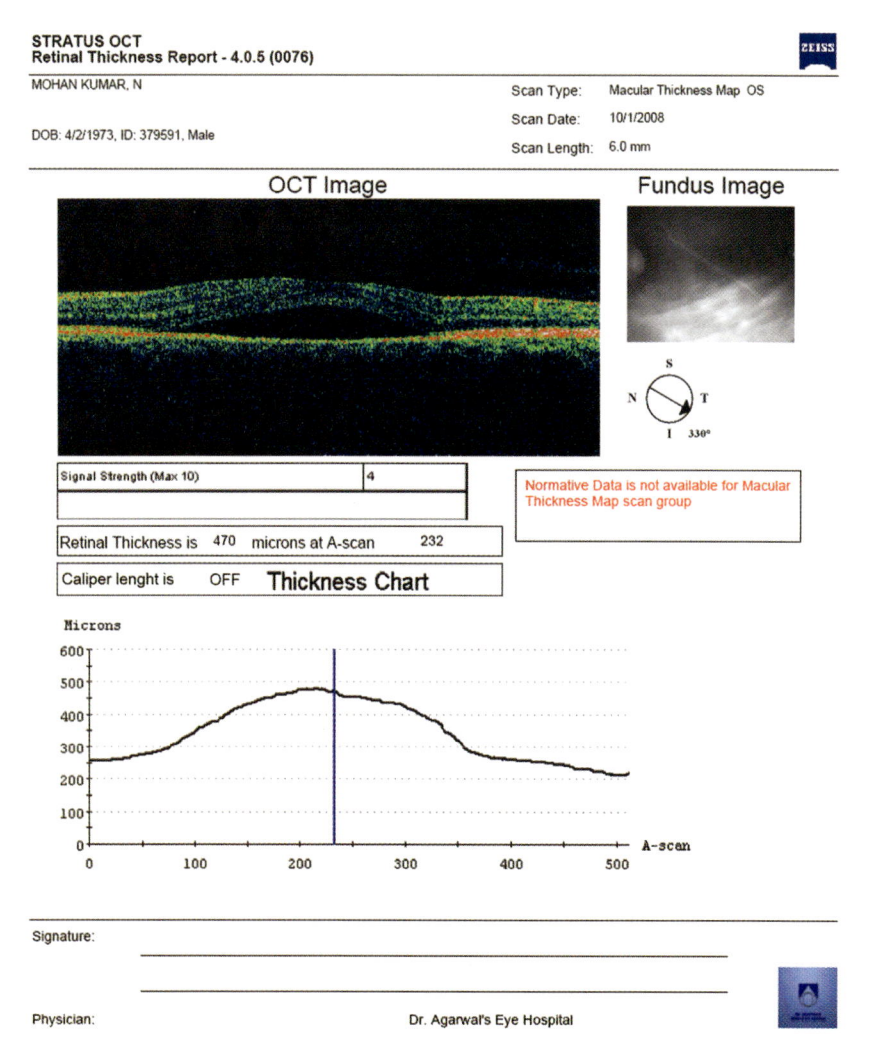

1. Give the diagnosis. Name the differential diagnosis.
2. What will be the criteria to do a laser treatment for this patient?
3. Name one contraindication for laser in this patient.
4. Give the soft sign on examination of this patient.
5. Where is the accumulation of fluid? Give the early and late FFA findings in this patient.

ANSWERS

1. The diagnosis of this patient is central serous retinopathy, CSR. The differential diagnosis is optic pit, macular detachment Choroidal tumours, SRNVM.
2. The criteria to treat this patient with laser will be multiple leaks on FFA, and presence of old CSR with loss of vision in the other eye.
3. The contraindication for doing laser will be leak that is present near the FAZ or within the FAZ.
4. A soft sign on examination is the presence of mild hypermetropia due to the detachment of sensory retina and its forward movement.
5. The fluid is accumulated between the sensory retina and the RPE. The early FFA finding is the presence of smoke stack or ink blot and the late FFA finding is the presence of mushroom or umbrella shape accumulation of dye.

QUESTION 41

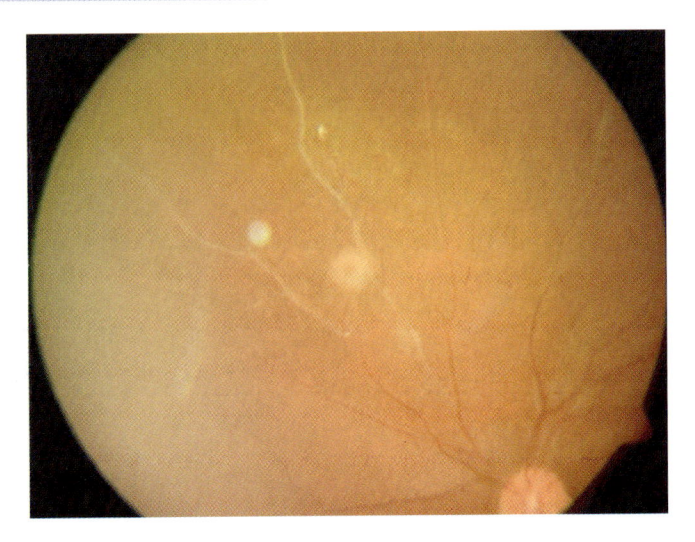

1. Describe the two diagnostic points seen in this clinical picture. Give your most likely diagnosis in a young adult male with a bilateral presentation.
2. Mention two complications that these patients will develop.
3. What will be the visual prognosis in this patient?
4. Where should the laser be done in this patient?
5. Presence of which association will call for a vitreoretinal surgery in this patient?

ANSWERS

1. Two diagnostic features seen in this patient are: vascular sheathing and new vessels elsewhere. The most likely diagnosis is Eales disease.
2. This patient can develop tractional retinal detachment and glaucoma secondary to rubeosis iridis.
3. The visual prognosis in these patients is good.
4. This patient needs a PRP if there is extensive involvement.
5. Presence of vitreous haemorrhage long standing with tractional retinal detachment will call for a vitreoretinal surgery.

QUESTION 42

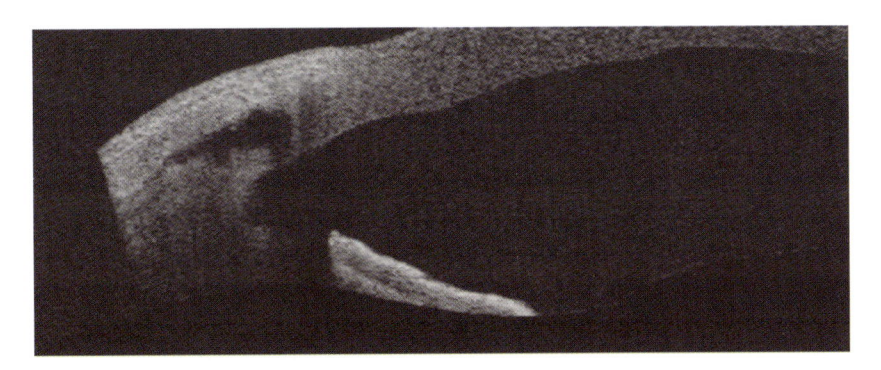

1. Explain the slide.
2. What is the laser wavelength used in anterior segment OCT?
3. Give one uses in glaucoma evaluation.
4. How much is the axial resolution of anterior segment OCT?

ANSWERS

1. This is picture of anterior segment OCT showing open angle with PI and Bleb with scleral flap
2. 1310 nm wavelength
3. It provides objective quantifiable measurement of the angle, even in opaque and edematous cornea
4. The axial resolution is 18 μm.

QUESTION 43

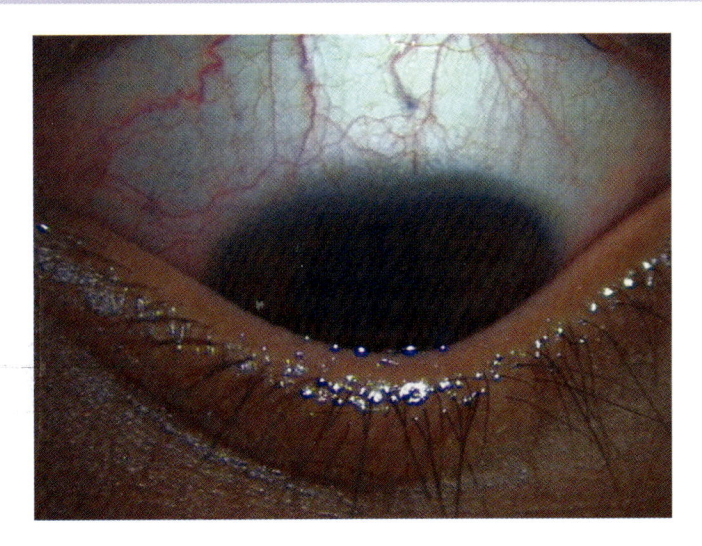

1. What is the sign shown in the picture? Describe the sign.
2. Name the sign seen in this patient on direct ophthalmoscopy.
3. What are the four systemic syndromes associated with this clinical condition?
4. Give the three grades on the basis of keratometry.
5. On the basis of slit-lamp examination how will you differentiate this thinning from pellucid marginal degeneration?

ANSWERS

1. The sign shown here is Munson's sign. It is the buldging or bowing of the lower lid when the patient is asked to look down.
2. On direct ophthalmoscopy there will be an oil droplet sign.
3. The systemic syndromes that can be associated with keratoconus are: Down's, Ehler Danlos, Turner's and Marfan's syndrome.
4. On basis of keratometry the keratoconus can be divided into mild less than 48D, moderate- 48-54D and severe more than 54D.
5. In case of PMO the thinning and ectatic points are different and in case of keratoconus, the thinning and ectatic points are at the same point.

QUESTION 44

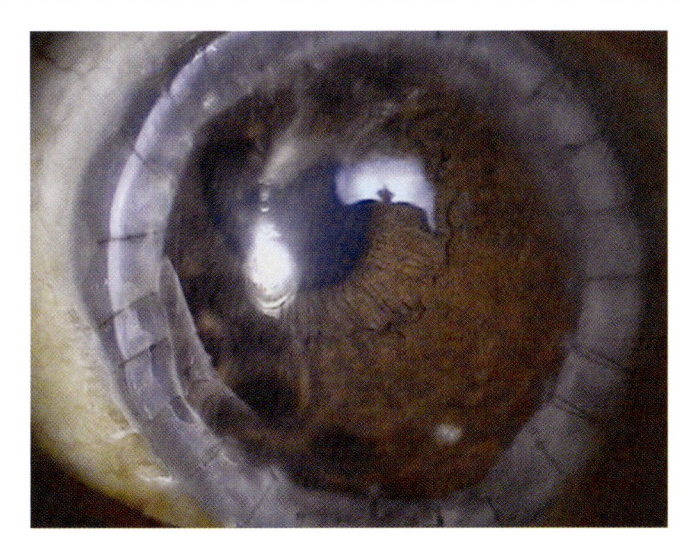

1. What is the surgery that has been done in this patient? What is the type of graft?
2. What are the two methods of suturing in keratoplasty, classify?
3. What is the commonest indication for the optical keratoplasty? Give the most favourable cases for penetrating keratoplasty?
4. What is a rare pupillary complication seen postoperatively?
5. How should the first sutures be placed? What are they called and in which order should they be placed with which suture material?

ANSWERS

1. This patient has undergone penetrating keratoplasty. It is a full thickness procedure with optical keratoplasty.
2. The two ways of suturing in PK are: indirect and direct. The direct is further classified into interrupted and continuous.
3. The commonest indication is Keratoconus. Cases with the best prognosis are keratoconus, corneal dystrophies and scarred corneas.
4. Urrets-Zavalia is the rare pupillary complication postop that consists of fixed dilated pupil.
5. The first sutures should be placed in the four quadrants. They are called cardinal sutures and the first one is at 12 then at 6 then at 3 followed by at 9 O' clock position. The suture material used commonly is 8/0 monofilament nylon or silk, which are removed at a later stage of the surgery.

QUESTION 45

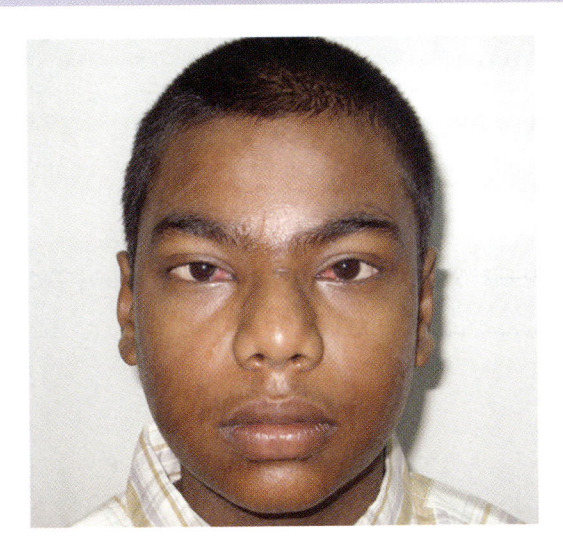

1. Which surgical procedure has been performed for this patient?
2. What are the types of strabismus operated with this type of surgery?
3. What is the relationship between the arc of contact with respect to recessions?
4. Name the other weakening muscle procedures done.

ANSWERS

1. A bimedial recession has been done on this patient.
2. Congenital esotropia, accommodative esotropia, nystagmus blockade syndrome are commonly operated with this type of surgery.
3. The recession procedure works as a weakening procedure as it decreases the arc of contact of the muscle.
4. The other weakening procedures carried out on muscles are: myectomy, myotomy, tenectomy, marginal myotomy and posterior fixation sutures.

QUESTION 46

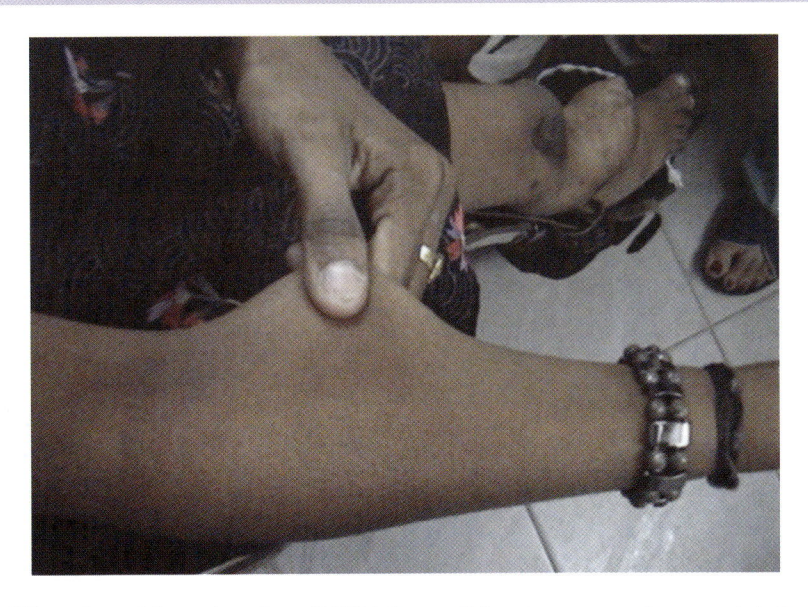

1. What does this patient have? Which condition is commonly associated with this sign?
2. Which other feature is present in the skin?
3. What are the ocular manifestations of the diseases?
4. What is the enzyme deficiency that is found in these patients and abnormality seen in the joints?

ANSWERS

1. The patient has hyperelasticity of the skin. Ehler-Danlos syndrome is commonly associated with hyperelasticity of the skin.
2. The other skin manifestation is Papyraceous skin, which bruises easily and heals with scarring.
3. The ocular manifestations are keratoconus, retinal detachment, high myopia and ectopia lentis commonly.
4. The enzyme deficient in the patients are procollagen lysyl hydroxylase that causes defective collagen production.

QUESTION 47

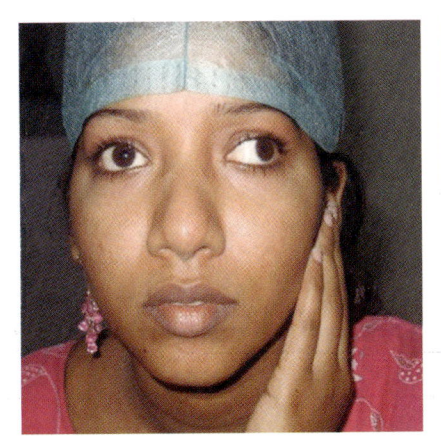

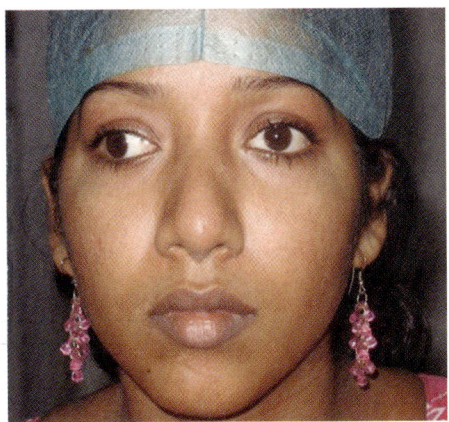

1. Give your diagnosis. Give two reasons for you answer.
2. How will you classify this type of strabismus?
3. Which test will determine the type of surgery to be done in this patient?
4. In terms of intermittent exotropia, what will be the surgical indications?
5. Will this patient have ARC? Give your reasons. What is the likely sensory adaptation in this patient?

ANSWERS

1. The patient has an alternating basic constant exotropia.
2. The exotropia are classified on the basis of Duane classification as follows: Basic exotropia, convergence insufficiency, divergence excess.
3. Patch test will show whether a unilateral or bilateral surgery should be done in this patient.
4. surgical indication intermittent exotropia are: squinting more than 50% of the time with loss of fusional control, loss of BSV, presence of constant exotropia of more than 15 prism diopters for distance or near.
5. No this patient will not have ARC, because the squint is a large angle exotropia that seems to alternate easily. The patient will have alternate eye suppression. ARC is seen with unilateral exotropia and intermittent exotropia.

QUESTION 48

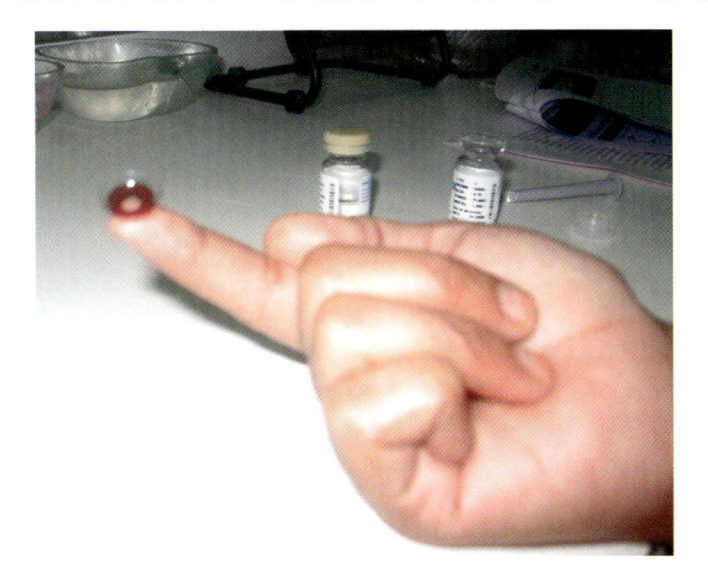

1. What is shown in the picture? What are the indications of its wear?
2. What is the contraindication of its uses?
3. What tests should be done in the eye before its use?
4. What is the most common disadvantage of soft contact lenses? What are the newer lenses that solve the problem and how?
5. What are the two important properties of extended wear lenses?

ANSWERS

1. The picture shoes a coloured soft cosmetic lens. The indications are cosmetic in scared and deformed eyes, therapeutic in ocular albinism and nystagmus.
2. Contraindications of use are: presence of dry eye, blephritis, ocular inflammations.
3. The following tests should be done before contact lens wear: tear strip measurement and examination, Schirrmers test, corneal surface slit-lamp and staining, corneal topography.
4. Presence of deposits are the most common disadvantages of a soft C.L. the new lenses that avoid this are the disposables as they are disposed before there can be an increase in deposits on their surface.
5. Extended wear lenses have high water content and high oxygen decay value – oxygen transmission to the cornea that is 6 times that of normal soft lenses.

QUESTION 49

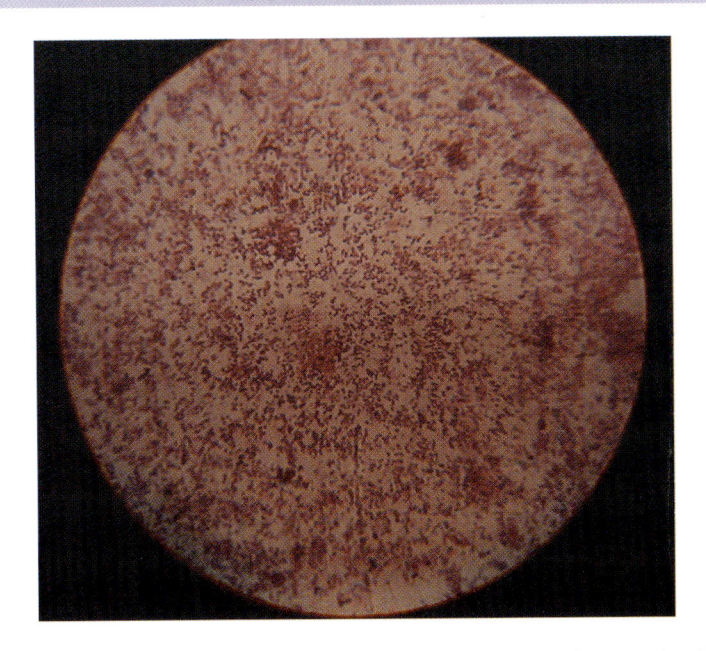

1. What is the typical location of the keratitis caused by this organism?
2. Mention the commonest type that will cause postsurgical endophthalmitis.
3. Give the culture characteristics of it's various types.
4. What is MRSA? Give its treatment.

ANSWERS

1. Marginal keratitis is commonly caused by this organism.
2. Staph epidermidis is most commonly responsible for postsurgical endophthalmitis.
3. They grow on nutrient agar, present as large circular smooth and shinny colonies, the colour of the colonies is golden yellow in case of Aureus, and in Staph epidermidis the color is white or pale yellow.
4. Methicillin resistance staphylococcus aureus is found in hospital acquired infection – nosocomial infections, it is treated with vancomycin eye drops.

QUESTION 50

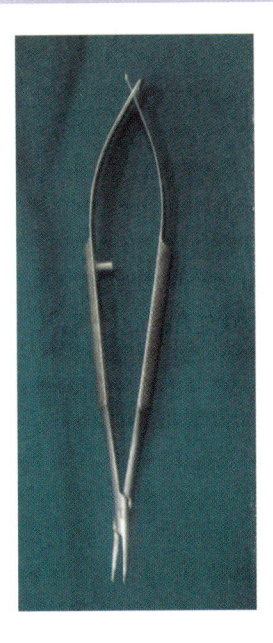

1. Identify this instrument.
2. Name two other types of the same instrument.
3. Which of the three will be used for extraocular procedures and why?
4. State the difference between this and the Castrovejo instrument.

ANSWERS

1. Barraquer needle holder.
2. Two other types of needle holders are: Castrovejo and Arruga.
3. The needle holder commonly used for extraocular procedures is called Arruga as it has larger and has a lock mechanism.
4. The Barraquer needle holder has curved end and the Castrovejo needle holder has straight ends.

Section 3

Question papers 51 to 75

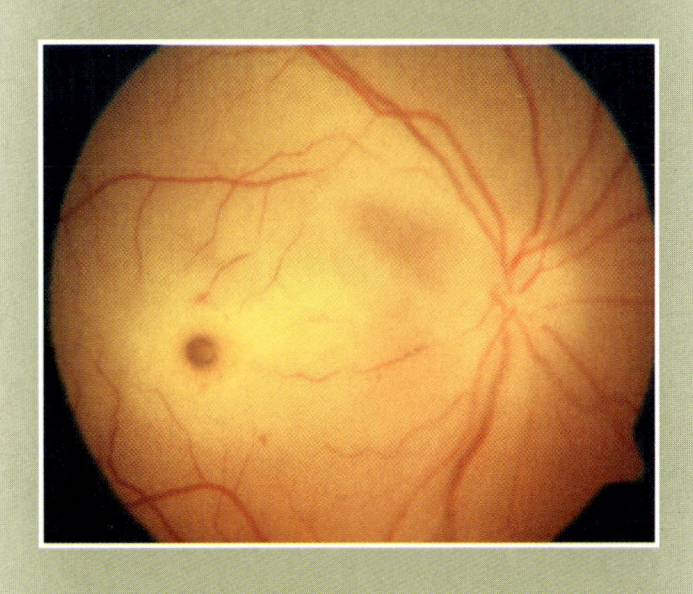

LID RETRACTION

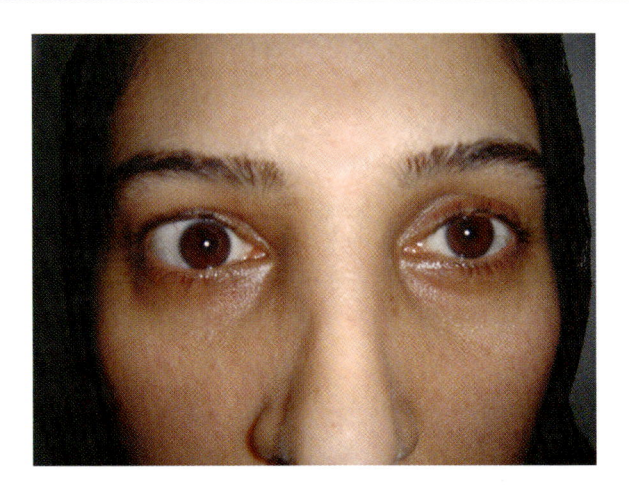

QUESTION 51

1. What does the right eye of this patient show? How will you differentiate this from pseudoretraction?
2. Give the commonest causes of pseudoretraction.
3. Give the two diagnostic signs in Dorsal midbrain syndrome and by what name is it known as? What are the associated features?
4. Classify the causes of lid retraction, stating commonest causes under each.
5. If surgery is planned then which is the commonly performed procedure in such cases?

ANSWERS

1. The right eye of this patient shows eye lid retraction. Pseudoretraction is ruled out by elevating the other side eyelid (appearing ptotic) and making that eye fixate. In case of pseudoretraction the retracted appearing eyelid assumes normal position once the contralateral eye is made to take up fixation.
2. Causes of pseudoretraction are: ptosis of the other eye, namely acquired apponeurotic type, facial palsy of the same side causing unopposed action of the levator and hemifacial spasm on the opposite side.
3. Two diagnostic signs of Dorsal midbrain syndrome are: light near papillary dissociation, gaze and convergence paralysis. These are called Collier's sign of Dorsal midbrain syndrome. Associated features are: vertical nystagmus, retraction nystagmus on upgaze, downgaze palsy, skew deviation and disturbances in fixation.
4. The causes of retraction can be classified as: Neurogenic, myogenic and mechanical. Common causes under each are:
   – *Neurogenic*: Dorsal midbrain syndrome
   – *Myogenic*: Graves ophthalmopathy
   – *Mechanical*: Myopia
5. Conjunctival mullerotomy is the most commonly performed surgical treatment.

QUESTION 52

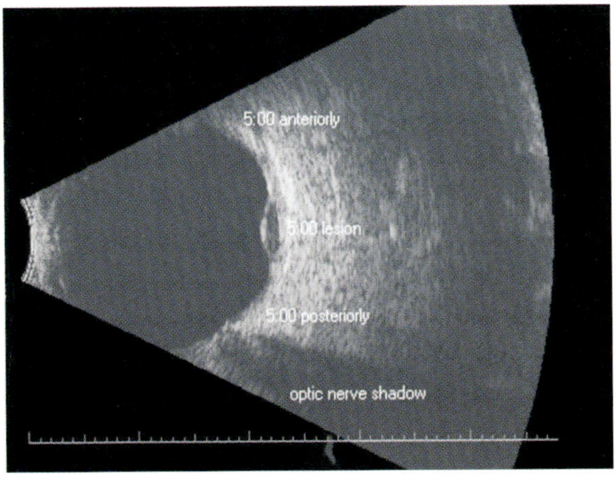
5:00 anteriorly
5:00 lesion
5:00 posteriorly
optic nerve shadow

1. What is the type of B scan taken here?
2. How should the probe be placed on the eye?
3. Which the commonest mode of B scan one and what are different modes that are available?
4. Explain the lesion seen above.

ANSWERS

1. The B scan taken here is the longitudinal mode of scan.
2. The probe should be placed perpendicular to the limbus on the eye.
3. The commonest mode of B scan done is the transverse mode. The different modes are: longitudinal, transverse, macular and axial.
4. The lesion seen is intraretinal and is a cystic lesion on the longitudinal mode as the radial extent of the lesion is seen well.

QUESTION 53

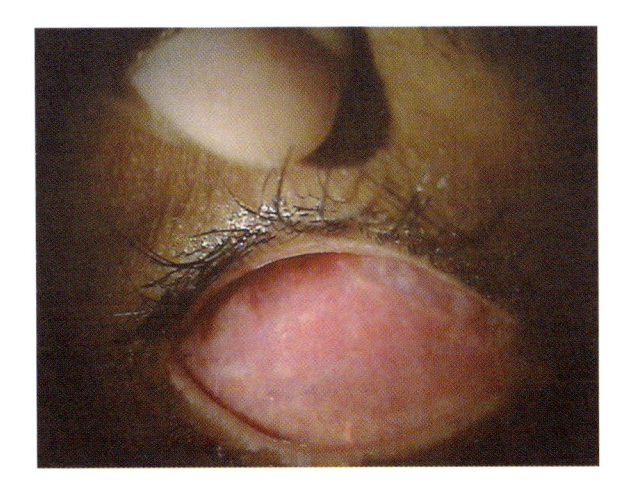

1. Describe the clinical picture with your diagnosis.
2. What are the two techniques of evisceration?
3. Mention the cosmetic advantages of this procedure.
4. Give the two types of this procedure and what is the difference between the two?
5. What dangerous disadvantage does this procedure have?

ANSWERS

1. The picture shows an anophthalmic socket with an implant.
2. The two techniques of evisceration are: evisceration with preservation of scleral button and without preservation of the scleral button.
3. The cosmetic advantage is lesser destruction of anatomical structures with good motility of the implant.
4. The two types of evisceration are: simple and frill evisceration. The frill evisceration involves preservation of 3 mm of sclera around the optic nerve and thus differs from simple evisceration that does not leave behind any sclera.
5. The most dangerous disadvantage is leaving behind a part of the intraocular tumour behind causing it's incomplete removal and hence a recurrence.

QUESTION 54

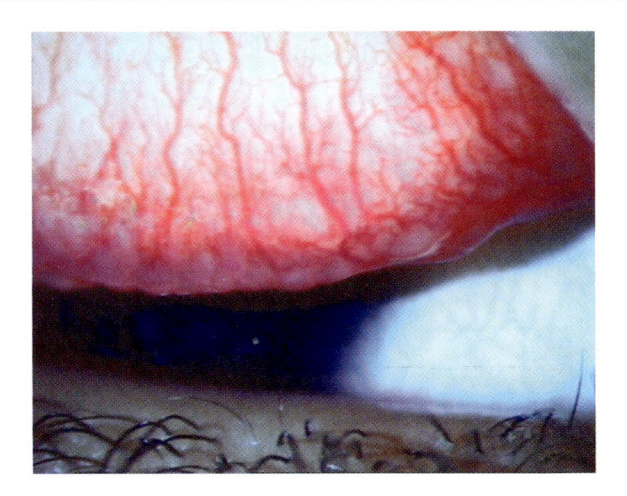

1. What is your diagnosis? Give the difference between macropapillae and giant papillae with respect to their size.
2. What type of secretion is associated with this condition if this is vernal catarrh?
3. What are the differential diagnoses of large papillae at the superior tarsal border?
4. What will the pathogenic difference between the reactions seen in vernal catarrh and in giant papillary conjunctivitis?
5. List the interventional treatments of the condition.

ANSWERS

1. The clinical photo shows Giant papillary conjunctival reaction. The macropapillae are 0.3 to 1 mm in size whereas the giant papillae are 1 to 2 mm in size.
2. Ropy white secretions are found when there is vernal catarrh.
3. Giant papillae at the superior tarsal border indicate long standing irritation as in the case of soft and RGP contact lens wear, loose suture material, ocular prosthesis and vernal catarrh.
4. The difference in the pathogenesis is that in vernal catarrh the reaction is IgE mediated and in Giant papillary conjunctivitis the reaction is *type 1 or type 4 hypersensitivity reaction*.
5. The interventional treatments consist of: shaving the papillary heads, applying cryotherapy to the hypertrophic areas, injection of subtarsal long acting steroids.

QUESTION 55

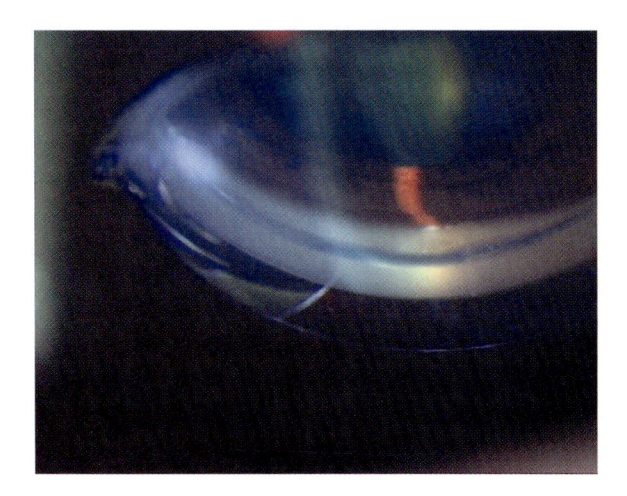

1. What investigation is being done here? What are the findings seen?
2. What will be your diagnosis and classify the causes?
3. What will the next step in management of this patient? Which drops will be used before the planned procedure?
4. What should be done by the examiner while using a Goldmann three mirror lens to see the angles better? How much pressure should be applied on the goniolens while carrying out the examination?
5. In postinflammatory angle closure, what are the diagnostic findings seen at the angles on gonioscopy?

ANSWERS

1. A gonioscopy is being performed. The angle structure is seen, with only the Schwalbe's line visible, the trabecular meshwork and the rest of the structures are not seen.
2. A diagnosis of angle closure glaucoma is made. The causes can be classified as primary angle closure and secondary angle closure with pulling or pushing mechanisms.
3. The next step should be Laser peripheral iridotomy. Pilocarpine should be instilled before the procedure to cause miosis and open the angle.
4. To see the angles better the mirror should be rotated towards the angle to be examined and the patient should be asked to look in the direction of the angle being studied. Enough pressure to cause equal distribution of the tear film meniscus between the lens and the anterior corneal surface should be applied. Also there should not be any Descemets folds on.
5. Gonioscopy of the angles in postinflammatory secondary angle closure will reveal the presence of fibrovascular membranes, PAS, pigments, inflammatory debris and angle new vessels in long standing cases.

QUESTION 56

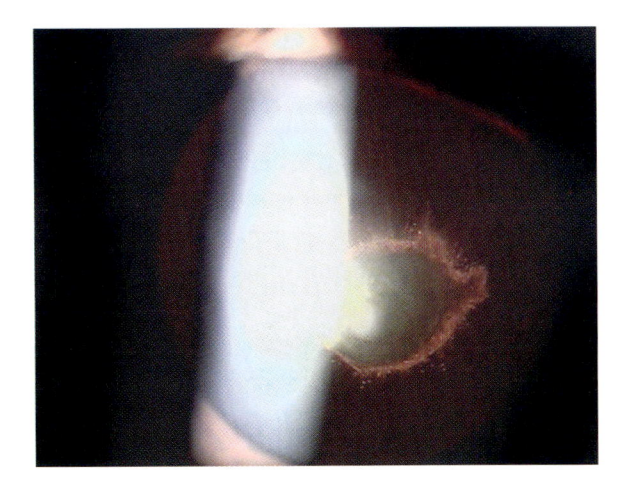

1. Give your diagnosis. Give two reasons for the diagnosis.
2. What are the other morphological types of congenital cataract?
3. What is the commonest type in congenital cases?
4. What surgical precaution should be taken at the time of phacoemulsification in this patient?
5. What are the anatomical differences between the anterior and the posterior pole of the lens?

ANSWERS

1. This shows the presence of posterior polar cataract. The site as well as the morphology is characteristic: the site is at the posterior pole of the lens, and the appearance is onion peel dense center with irregular borders.
2. The other morphological types of congenital cataract are: punctate, zonular, fusiform, nuclear, coronary and anterior capsular.
3. Commonest type in congenital cases is lamellar/zonular cataract.
4. At the time of phacoemulsification, this patient should undergo good hydrodelination but hydrodissection should be avoided.
5. The anterior pole has a thicker capsule, the capsule of the lens in thin at the posterior pole. The cells of the lens are cuboidal at the anterior pole whereas at the posterior pole they tend to be columnar.

QUESTION 57

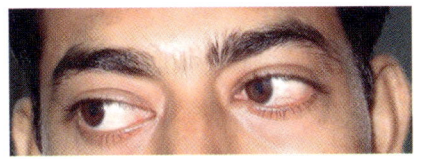

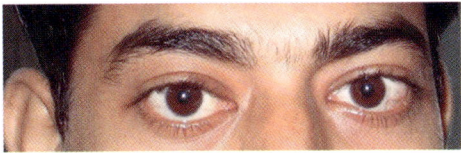

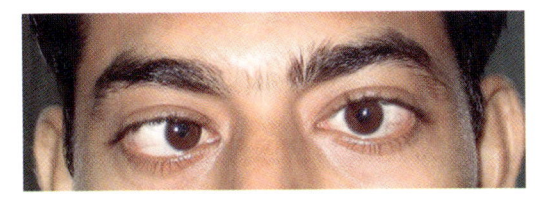

1. Give your diagnosis. Which are the two surgical procedures that can be performed in this patient?
2. State the difference between the two surgical procedures.
3. What will be the differential diagnosis of this patient?
4. What will be most common 4 causes in this young patient if it is an acquired palsy?
5. If the palsy is associated with pain then could be the causes.

ANSWERS

1. This patient has left sixth nerve palsy. The two surgical procedures that can be performed are: Hummelshliem procedure and Jensons procedure.
2. In Hummelshliem procedure – the lateral halves of the superior and inferior recti are disinserted and attached to the lateral rectus. MR recession is also done.

   In Jensen's procedure: It is not disinserted, the muscles of superior, inferior lateral recti are split lengthways. Lateral half superior rectus and superior part of lateral rectus is tied with a nonabsorbable suture and likewise inferior part of lateral rectus and lateral part of inferior rectus are tied.
3. The differential diagnosis is: Duane syndrome, medial wall fracture with muscle entrapment of the medial rectus, thyroid ophthalmopathy, and myasthenia gravis.
4. Acquired sixth nerve palsy occurring in a young adult should be due to: trauma, tumour, postviral or ischemic mononeuropathy.
5. Painful sixth nerve palsy should arouse the suspicion of: Gradenigo's syndrome, petrous apex syndrome, orbital apex syndrome, cavernous sinus syndrome.

QUESTION 58

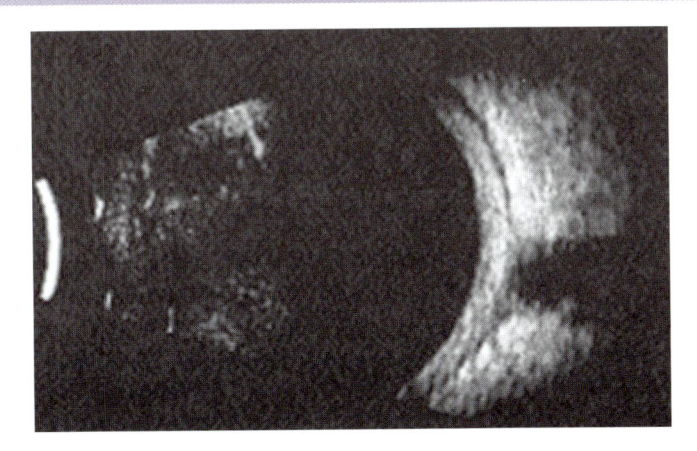

1. What does the B scan show? What is the sign called and which clinical condition is diagnosed?
2. What will be the associated posterior segment or retinal findings in this patient?
3. How will you classify anterior scleritis?
4. Which systemic association with this clinical condition?
5. What is pulse therapy, what is the drug used, why is it given?

ANSWERS

1. The B scan shows thickening of the posterior layers of the sclera, the sign is called inverted T sign; it is diagnostic of posterior scleritis.
2. The retina can show disc and macular oedema, retinal exudative detachment and posterior segment can also show Choroidal folds, detachment and uveal effusion syndrome.
3. Anterior scleritis is classified as nodular, diffuse and necrotising.
4. Systemic association associated with posterior scleritis are: rheumatoid arthritis, Ankylosing Spondylitis, Reiger's syndrome, polyarteritis nodosa and systemic lupus erythematosis.
5. Pulse therapy is the intravenous use of immunosuppressive, the drug used is intravenous methylprednisolone. *It is given so as to decrease the dependence on steroids and avoid the complications of long-term steroid use.*

QUESTION 59

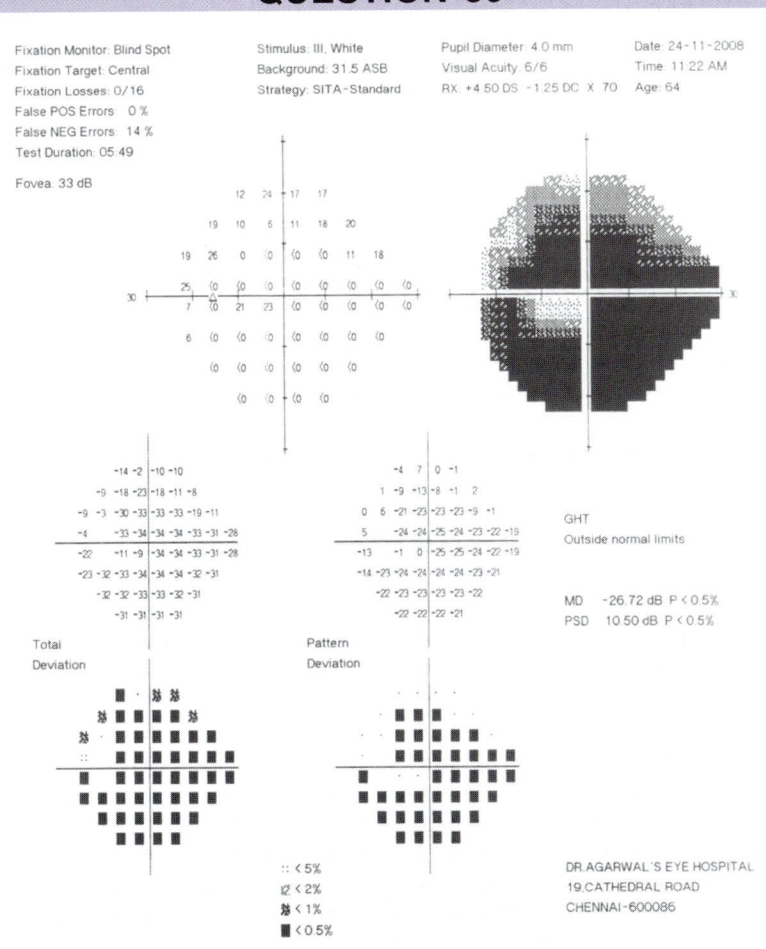

Fixation Monitor: Blind Spot
Fixation Target: Central
Fixation Losses: 0/16
False POS Errors: 0 %
False NEG Errors: 14 %
Test Duration: 05:49

Fovea: 33 dB

Stimulus: III, White
Background: 31.5 ASB
Strategy: SITA-Standard

Pupil Diameter: 4.0 mm
Visual Acuity: 6/6
RX: +4.50 DS -1.25 DC X 70

Date: 24-11-2008
Time: 11:22 AM
Age: 64

GHT
Outside normal limits

MD -26.72 dB P < 0.5%
PSD 10.50 dB P < 0.5%

Total Deviation

Pattern Deviation

:: < 5%
& < 2%
※ < 1%
■ < 0.5%

DR.AGARWAL'S EYE HOSPITAL
19.CATHEDRAL ROAD
CHENNAI-600086

1. What does the visual field show? What are the fibres left intact in this field?
2. What will be the differential diagnosis?
3. What should be the next visual field ordered in this patient, and with which target size?
4. What should be seen on the above ordered field, what is its clinical significance?
5. In retinitis pigmentosa, what is the other name given to this type of vision field loss?

ANSWERS

1. The visual field shows the presence of tubular visual field loss. The fibres that are intact are the papillomacular bundle fibres.
2. The differential diagnosis are: advanced stage of glaucoma, retinitis pigmentosa, PRP,
3. The next type of visual field ordered should be the macular threshold with target 5.
4. If there is splitting of the macular fields or more than two quadrants are involved then an intraocular surgery is contraindicated (because of the chance of Wipe out syndrome).
5. Retinitis pigmentosa causes a ring scotoma to develop or a double ring scotoma to develop.

QUESTION 60

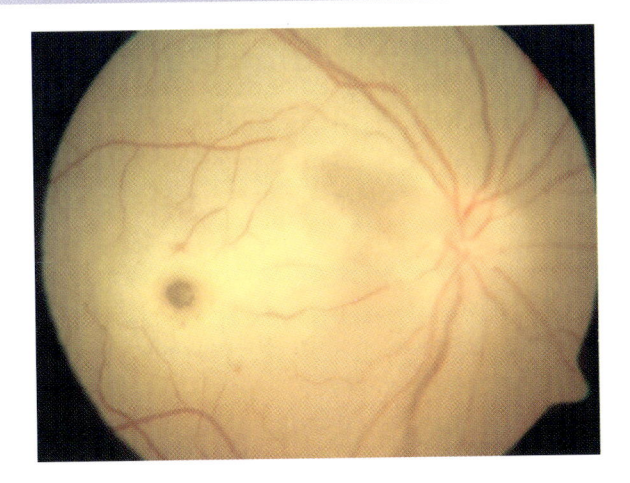

1. Give your diagnosis and 3 points in favour of the same.
2. How will this patient present and what will be the pupillary reaction in this patient?
3. What are the types of carotid artery emboli, which is the most dangerous one and why?
4. What are the ocular causes of arterial obstruction?
5. Give the features of vision loss in Amaurosis Fugax.

ANSWERS

1. This fundus picture appears to be that of CRAO. Three points in favour of this arc: retinal oedema indicated by white reflex; the arterial vessels are narrow and the foveal area shows a cherry red spot.
2. The patients will present with sudden profound vision loss and the pupil will show Marcus-Gunn pupil reaction.
3. The types of carotid artery emboli are: cholesterol, calcific and fibrinoplatelet. The calcific emboli are the most dangerous as they cause permanent occlusion and are difficult to dislodge.
4. Ocular causes of arterial obstruction are: arteritis, atheroma, raised intraocular pressure and rarely retinal migraine.
5. Amaurosis Fugax is characterised by transient vision loss that is painless, unilateral, and occurs from top to bottom. It also recovers in the same direction.

QUESTION 61

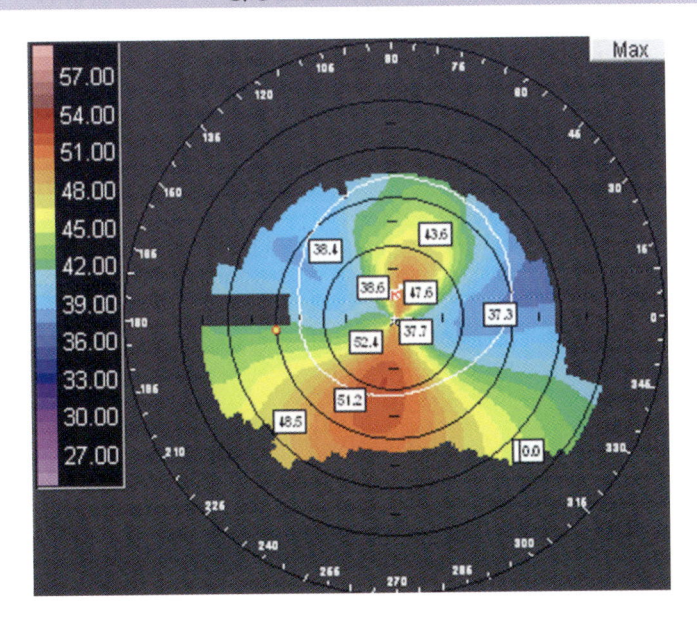

1. What is the principle of orbscan?
2. Is it with the rule or against the rule astigmatism in the given orbscan.
3. Which type of scale is shown in the picture?
4. What are surgical treatments for astigmatism?
5. What is Ruiz procedure?

ANSWERS

1. Three dimensional slit scan technology.
2. This orbscan shows with the rule astigmatism.
3. Absolute scale has been shown.
4. Transverse incision, arcuate incision, Limbal relaxing incision, Astigmatic lasik, relaxing incision with compression suture, corneal wedge resection.
5. Deep horizontal keratotomy incisions are made with a guarded diamond blade in step ladder configuration, along the axis of the steepest corneal meridian. Each set of horizontal incisions is flanked by two adjacent radial incisions.

QUESTION 62

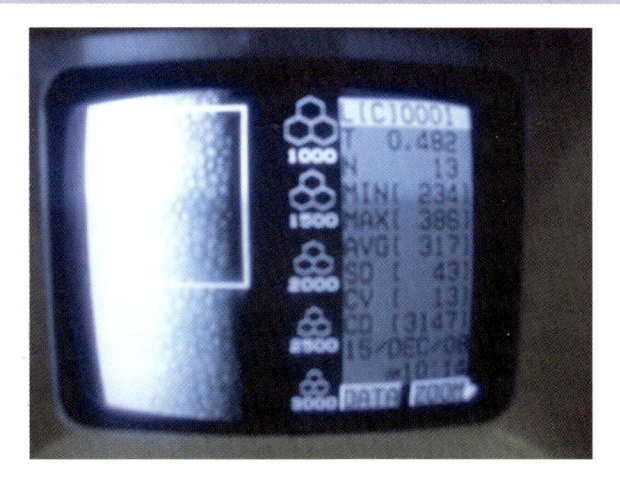

1. What is this instrument and state its principle? What is responsible for specular reflection?
2. Name the zones of reflection occurring at the time of examination with this instrument.
3. What are the two types of specular microscopy? Which two characteristics of corneal cells are studied with specular microscopy?
4. What is wide field specular microscopy? Give its two advantages.
5. Name the indices used to take the measurements?
6. How is coefficient of variation calculated and give its significance and normal value?

ANSWERS

1. This is the specular microscope. Its principle is that it utilizes the light reflected from the optical interface of tissue for forming the image. The difference between the refractive index of the endothelial cells and the aqueous humour causes specular reflection on a flat surface.
2. The Zones of images formation are :
   - Zone 1 – epithelium/lens coupling fluid.
   - Zone 2 – corneal stroma
   - Zone 3 – corneal endothelium
   - Zone 4 – aqueous humour.
3. Contact and noncontact type of specular microscopy. Corneal thickness and Corneal cell shape are studied well.
4. Wide field specular utilizes high speed oscillating mirrors so that 800 microns of diameter area is viewed as a single field. The two advantages are: (a) This is a 10 to 15 times larger field, (b) The image resolution and magnification are also higher with this instrument.
5. The indices used are:MAX: maximum cell area, MIN: minimum cell area, NUM: number of cells counted/seen, CD: cell density, SD: standard density, CV: coefficient of variation, AVE: average cell area.
6. CV is calculated by SD/AVE. The normal value should not exceed 0.25. An increase in CV shows polymegathism.

QUESTION 63

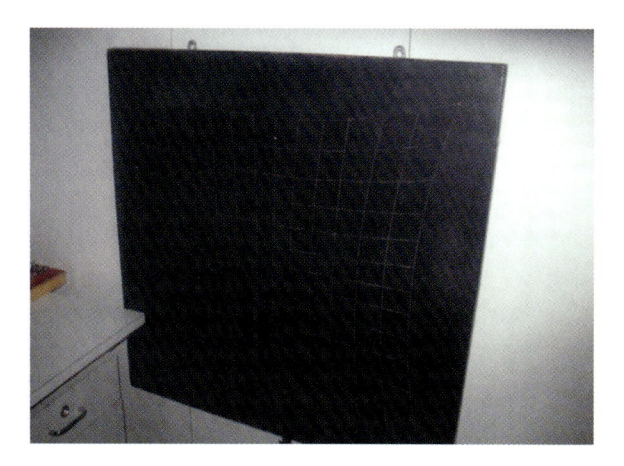

1. What test can be done with this instrument? Name two other tests that be used for the same purpose.
2. What type of squint will you recommend this test for? Should this test be repeated once again after an interval of few days? Give reason for your answer.
3. What is the angle subtended by each of the squares? How many degrees do the smaller and the larger square represent and what do they test?
4. What distance does the patient sit from the screen, what colour light does the patient hold and what colour is placed in front of the fixing eye?
5. What is the principle of this test? How does it differ from the diplopia principle?

ANSWERS

1. Hess charting is carried out with this instrument. The Less screen test and Lancaster red green test are the other two tests that can be done.
2. All Incomitant squints especially paralytic should be tested on this. Yes, Hess charting should be repeated after an interval of 3 to 6 months. It is useful for noting the progress of the disease – prognostic feature.
3. The angle subtended by the squares is 5 degrees. The small square represents central 15 degrees and the larger square is 30 degrees. The small square measures the normal range of versions and the larger square denotes extreme gaze positions.
4. The patient is seated 50 cm away and holds the green light in the hand. The fixing eye is the eye with red glass in front of it.
5. The principle of this text is the haploscopic principle. The haploscopic principle differs from the diplopia principle in that, here two test objects are given to the patient at the same time and then the patient has to superimpose them.

QUESTION 64

STRATUS OCT
Retinal Thickness Report - 4.0.5 (0076)

LALITHA AMMAL, R

DOB: 9/29/1948, ID: 027780, Female

Scan Type: Macular Thickness Map OD
Scan Date: 9/29/2008
Scan Length: 6.0 mm

OCT Image

Fundus Image

Signal Strength (Max 10): 5

Normative data is not available for macular thickness map scan group

Retinal Thickness is 208 microns at A-scan 260
Caliper Length is OFF

Thickness Chart

1. What does the OCT show? What are the common causes?
2. How can an early membrane be appreciated on ophthalmoscopy? What are the fundus features of a membrane present at the macula?
3. What are types of surgeries possible in this patient?
4. What are instruments used?
5. How is the membrane stained and which is the best method of membrane removal and why?

ANSWERS

1. The OCT shows presence of an epiretinal membrane. The common causes are diabetic retinopathy, exudative ARMD secondary to SRNVM, trauma, cellophane maculopathy and postphotocoagulation, RD surgery or cryo.
2. An early membrane is detected by using a Red free light on ophthalmoscopy. Retinal characteristics of a membrane are fine striae on the retinal surface with traction on the retinal vessels causing stretching and straightening of the retinal vessels.
3. Three types of surgeries that are possible one segmentation, delamination and peeling.
4. The instruments used are diamond dusted forceps and membrane pick.
5. The membrane is stained with Trypan blue and the peeling is the best method of removal as it causes removal of the membrane in totality.

QUESTION 65

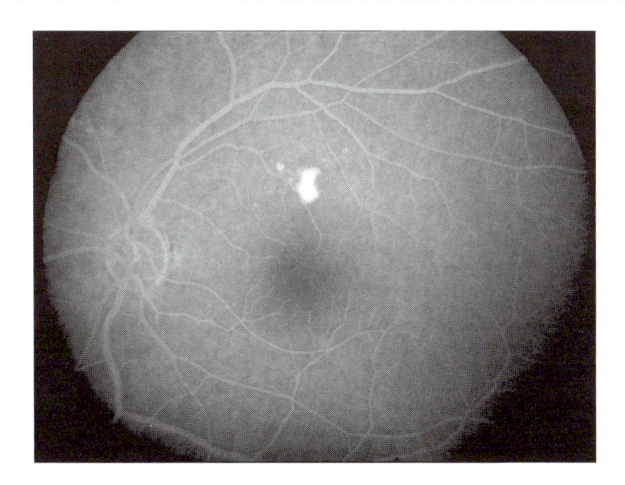

1. Describe the FFA picture. Which phase has it been taken? Give the common diagnosis.
2. What are the causes? Where is the fluid collected?
3. What will be the early and the late FFA findings?
4. What are the consequences in this patient?

ANSWERS

1. There is a focal well-circumscribed area of hyperfluorescence of the FFA taken in the late phase. Localised PED is the probable diagnosis.
2. Causes of PED are: exudative ARMD, SRNVM secondary to trauma, tumours, and high myopias. The fluid is collected in the sub RPE space between the RPE and the Bruchs membrane.
3. Early FFA shows hyperfluorescence and pooling of the dye, while the late phase shows well-circumscribed margins of the detachment.
4. The following are the consequences:
   – There can be spontaneous resolution
   – Spread of the RPE detachment causing detachment of the sensory retina
   – Tear or break in the RPE layer.

QUESTION 66

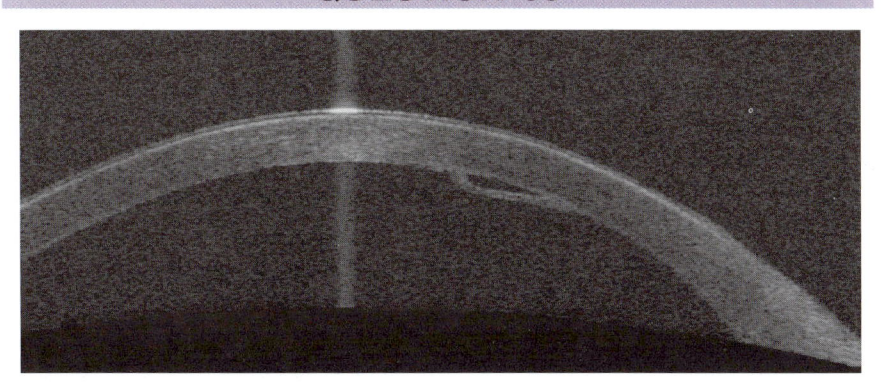

1. What is seen in this Figure?
2. What is the surgical treatment? Name 2 commonly practised methods?
3. Two uses of anterior segment OCT in post-lasik cases.
4. What is the resolution of UBM and that of the anterior segment OCT?

ANSWERS

1. Localized descemets detachment is seen here.
2. Surgical treatment is as follows: (a) Putting an air bubble in anterior chamber which pushes descemets on to the cornea, (b) Suture from descemets membrane tear area to full thickness of cornea.
3. Flap measurements, residual bed thickness can be measured postoperatively by using the anterior segment OCT.
4. 50 μm is the resolution of the UBM and 80 μm is the anterior segment OCT resolution.

QUESTION 67

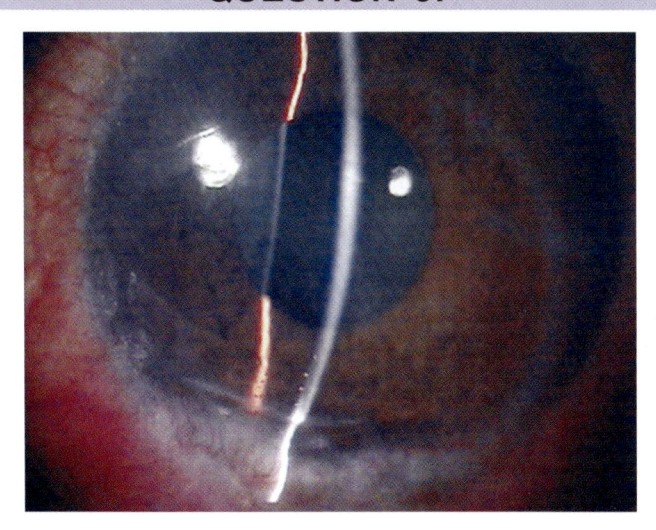

1. What type of keratitis does this patient have? Give two characteristic findings.
2. What are the systemic diseases associated with this?
3. How will you differentiate this condition from Moorens ulcer?
4. What are the diseases causing involvement of the peripheral part of the cornea?
5. How will you manage this patient medically and surgically?

ANSWERS

1. This patient has peripheral ulcerative keratitis. Two characteristic features are: crescent shaped peripheral infiltration and associated scleritis.
2. Systemic diseases associated with this are: rheumatoid arthritis. Systemic lupus erythematosis, Wegners granulomatosis and relapsing polychondritis.
3. Moorens ulcer does not cause scleritis and scleral involvement.
4. Peripheral cornea is affected in: marginal keratitis caused by – *Staphylococcus*, phlyctenular keratitis, rosacea keratitis, riboflavin deficiency, peripheral ulcerative keratitis, exposure keratopathy and keratitis associated with lid and lash abnormalities.
5. This patient should be started on topical and oral high dose steroids. Cytotoxic drugs like cyclophosphamide, azathioprines and methotrexate can also be started. The surgical treatment will be penetrating or lamellar keratoplasty.

QUESTION 68

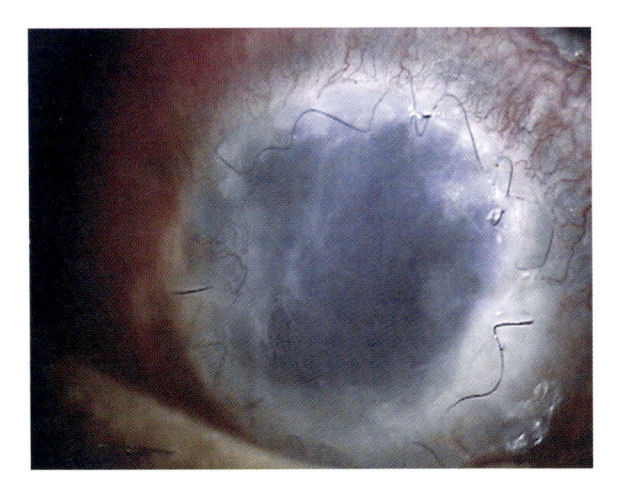

1. Describe the clinical finding. Give the likely diagnosis in this patient.
2. What do you mean by the term primary donor failure? Mention its causes.
3. What are the three types of rejection and give their important underlying feature?
4. How will you manage this patient, answer with respect to clinical tests investigation and treatment?

ANSWERS

1. The clinical picture shows the presence of a totally opaque graft with loose continuous sutures and vascularizations at the periphery of the graft and limbus 360 degrees. The conjunctiva is congested and the details of the anterior chamber are not seen. The likely diagnosis: graft failure.
2. Primary donor failure occurs from the first postop day and it is due to faulty donor material causing a thickened oedematous graft with DM folds on the very next day.
3. The three types of rejection are epithelial characterised by an elevated line, stromal characterised by Krachmer spots and endothelial characterised by Khodadoust line.
4. The clinical examination should include Va, IOP, dry eye assessment. Investigation should be ultrasound of the eye, conjunctival swab and staining. The patient treatment will be topical steroids, antiglaucoma medication and surgery will consist of full thickness penetrating keratoplasty.

QUESTION 69

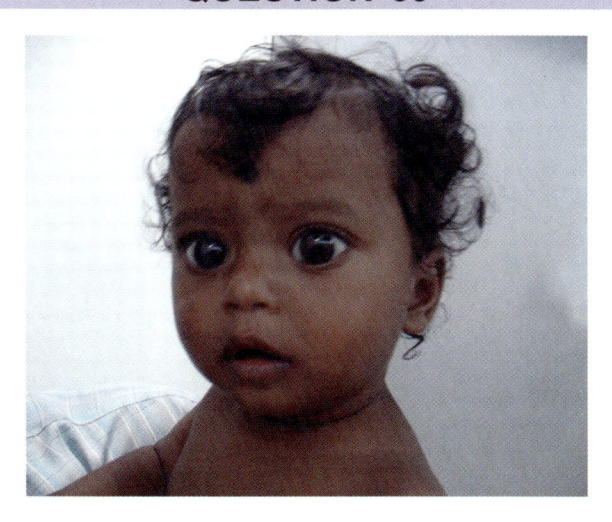

1. What does this child have? What is the common differential diagnosis?
2. What are the parameters that should be studied when this child is posted for examination under anaesthesia?
3. What are the parameters of the corneal size to be diagnosed as megalocornea? What is the inheritance pattern?
4. What is the most common form? Mention the associated ocular defects that can be present.

ANSWERS

1. The child has megalocornea. The child should be differentiated from congenital glaucoma.
2. The parameters to be recorded are: intraocular pressure, size of the cornea vertical and horizontal, microscopy of the anterior segment, gonioscopy, cycloplegic refraction, fundus picture with optic nerve head description and, A scan.
3. The parameters for megalocornea to be diagnosed are a size of greater than 13 mm in an infant and 12 mm in the newborn. The condition is X linked recessive.
4. The most common form is anterior megalophthalmos and it is associated with lens subluxation, iris transillumination defects and ectopic pupil.

QUESTION 70

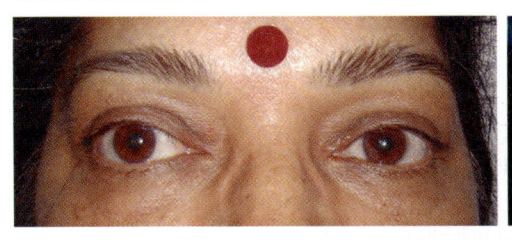

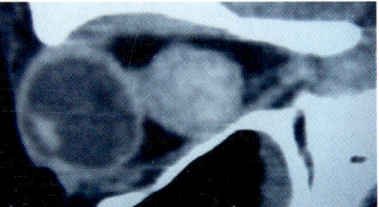

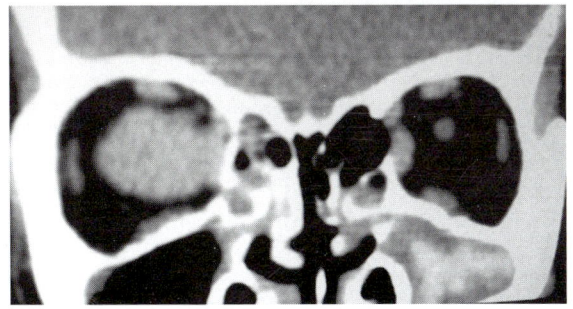

1. What does the clinical photograph show? Give differential diagnosis.
2. What does the CT scan show? What is the most likely diagnosis?
3. Give the characteristic pictures on CT of glioma and meningiomas of the optic nerve.
4. What would have been the clinical picture if the tumour was at the orbital apex? Comment on the pupillary reaction and vision status of the patient in such cases of orbital apex involvement.
5. What can the fundus picture show in this patient?

ANSWERS

1. The clinical photo shows the presence of unilateral axial proptosis. The common differentials are: thyroid eye disease, optic nerve meningioma, cavernous haemangioma, optic nerve glioma.
2. The CT scan shows presence of an intraconal mass along the optic nerve. The most likely diagnosis is cavernous haemangioma.
3. Optic nerve gliomas have a characteristic fusiform enlargement of the optic nerve and meningioma of the optic nerve show calcifications with thickening of the nerve.
4. Tumour situated at the optic apex would not have caused significant proptosis and have caused an afferent pupillary defect and vision loss.
5. The fundus will show presence of chorioretinal folds and optic disc oedema if the tumour compresses the posterior part of the globe.

QUESTION 71

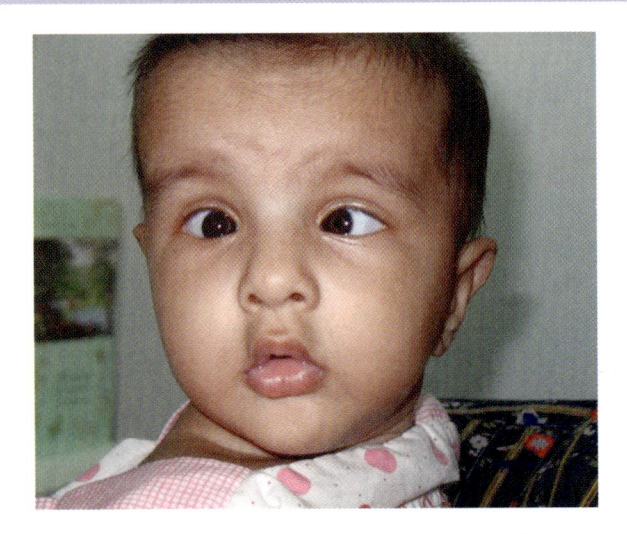

1. What does this child have? Give its differential diagnosis.
2. What are the associated features that should be looked for in this child?
3. At what age should the child undergo surgery? Give two reasons.
4. What are the surgical outcomes in this child? Which of them are acceptable and which are nonacceptable?
5. What is the advantage of posterior fixation sutures over large medial rectus recessions?

ANSWERS

1. This child has essential infantile esotropia/congenital esotropia. The differential diagnosis is: congenital 6th nerve palsy, nystagmus blockade syndrome, accommodative esotropia, Duane retraction syndrome type 1.
2. The associated features that this child should be examined for are: latent nystagmus, DVD, primary inferior oblique overaction and asymmetric OKN.
3. The child should undergo surgery before 2 years of age. Sometimes even in the first year. The reasons are that early surgery provides good functional results with respect to binocular vision and also that secondary changes in the tenons and muscle sheaths are avoided making it easy for the surgeon and results more predictable.
4. There are four surgical outcomes possible: microtropia and subnormal binocular vision, both of these are acceptable results. The others are small and large angle residual esotropia or consecutive exotropia. The large angle results are not acceptable and require a resurgery.
5. Posterior fixation sutures have lesser chances of causing consecutive exotropia than large recession of the medial rectus.

QUESTION 72

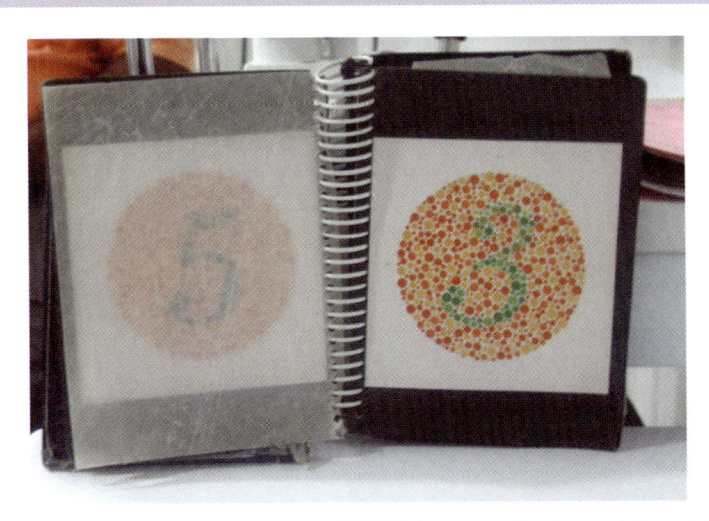

1. What are these plates shown here? Which type of colour vision defect due they largely identify?
2. What are isochromatic charts? Give another example of an isochromatic chart and which colour blindness does it identify.
3. What test is used in toxic optic neuropathy with a characteristic pattern?
4. Which conditions should undergo red green colour perimetry and what is central relative scotoma?
5. What colours are affected in the retinal diseases? What is the inheritance in congenital form?

ANSWERS

1. The plates here are of Ishihara charts. They largely identify red green abnormalities.
2. Isochromatic charts are lithographic plates that have a number represented by dots, set amidst dots of various similar confusing tints. Hardy R and Ritter are also isochromatic plates that mainly detect blue-yellow blindness.
3. The Farnsworth Munsell 100 hue test is used in toxic optic neuropathy.
4. Red green perimetry should be carried out in toxic optic neuropathies like alcohol and smoking and also in retrobulbar neuritis. The defect achieved by red green perimetry that disappears on blue or ordinary perimetry is called central relative scotoma.
5. Retinal diseases give rise to blue-yellow colour vision defects. The inheritance of congenital colour blindness is X-linked recessive.

QUESTION 73

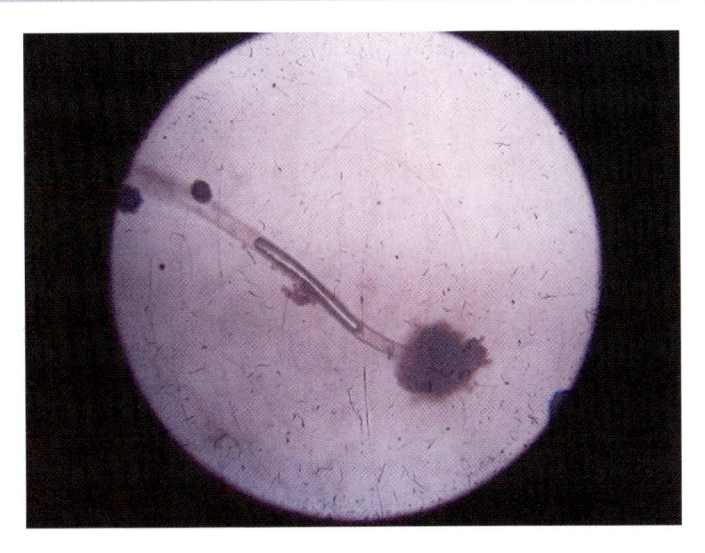

1. What is the staining used? Name the other methods of staining this organism.
2. Identify the organism, give your reasons.
3. What type of keratitis will this cause?
4. What are the culture plates that can be used?
5. Give the culture characteristics.

ANSWERS

1. The stain used is Lactophenol cotton blue. The other methods are KOH, Giemsa and Grocotts methanamine silver.
2. The organism is Aspergillus. The reasons are: presence of conidiophores which is a swollen end with spores and radiating conidia. The hyphae are branching and septate.
3. This will cause central suppurative ulcerative keratitis.
4. The culture plates that can be used are: Sabroud agar with gentamicin, thioglycolate broth and liquid brain heart infusion broth.
5. The culture of A. Fumigatus will show white followed by green moulds appearing in few hours and the A. Niger will show black colonies.

QUESTION 74

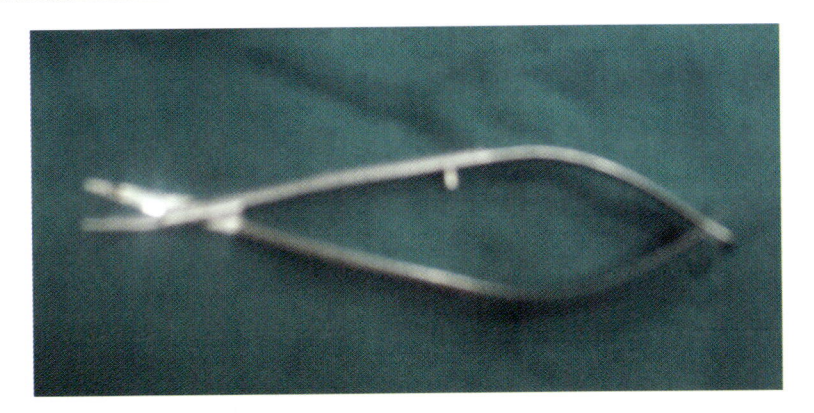

1. Identify this instrument.
2. What are the types of scissors available? What is the use of having its different angles?
3. Which is the scissor used in cutting fine structures like the anterior lens capsule?
4. Which is an iris scissor and mention its differences from other tissue cutting scissors?

ANSWERS

1. This instrument is Castrovejo corneoscleral scissors.
2. The types are straight, right angled and left angled. The right and the left angled are specially designed so that the cutting of the host button during PK is made easy.
3. Vannas scissors is a fine tissue cutting scissor.
4. DeWeckers scissors is an iris cutting scissor and it differs from the other scissors in that it has a spring action and it has right angled blades that cross each other.

QUESTION 75

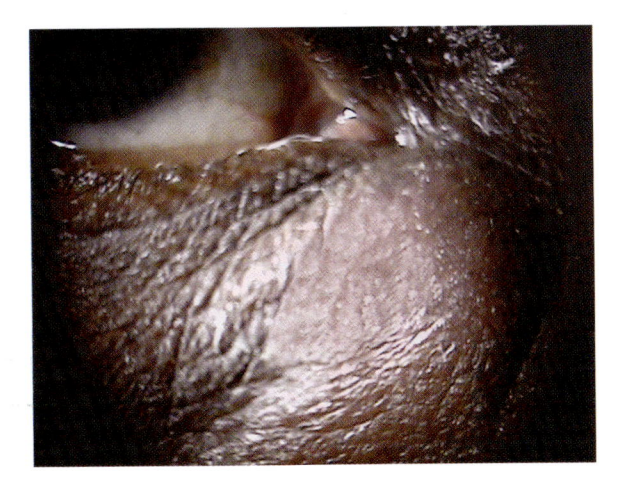

1. What is the diagnosis? How will you differentiate a congenital dacryocele from encephalocoele?
2. What is a soft stop and what is a hard stop, give their significance?
3. What are the three main causes of epiphora?
4. What will be findings in primary Jones dye test and in secondary Jones dye test if the obstruction is in the NLD?
5. What is the cause of encysted mucocoele? What investigation should be carried out in case of a palpable mass?

ANSWERS

1. This clinical picture looks like a lacrimal mucocoele. The congenital cases are differentiated from encephalocoele by the presence of a pulsatile swelling that is felt above the medial canthal tendon.
2. A soft stop is felt during lacrimal probing when there is soft tissue felt between the probe and the lacrimal bone. The soft stop is due to cannalicular obstruction. The hard stop is when the probe hits the bone directly after entering the lacrimal sac. It indicates that the cannalicular system is patent and the block is in the NLD.
3. The three main causes of epiphora are: excessive secretion, functional loss of drainage and obstructive cause.
4. Primary Jones test will be negative and Secondary Jones test will be positive if the NLD obstruction is partial.
5. Encysted mucocoeles are caused by mucosal stenosis of the sac wall or stricture of the cannaliculus. In case a mass is palpable then dacryocystography and CT scan should be ordered.

Section 4

Question papers 76 to 100

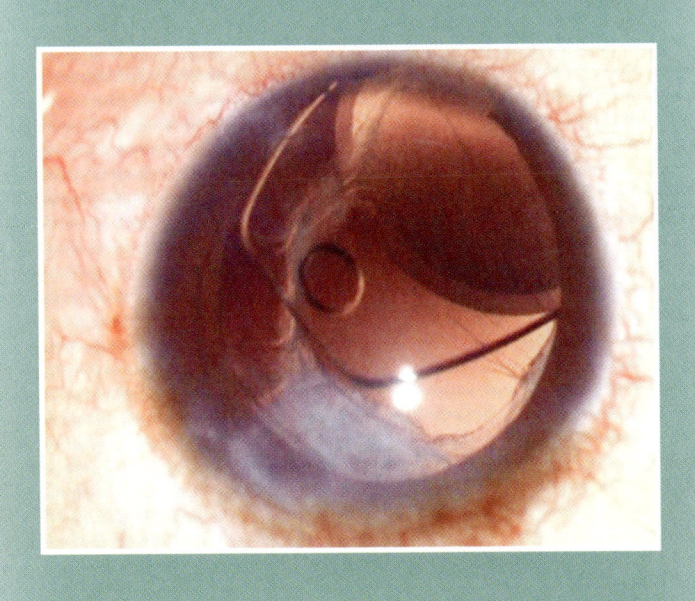

PTOSIS

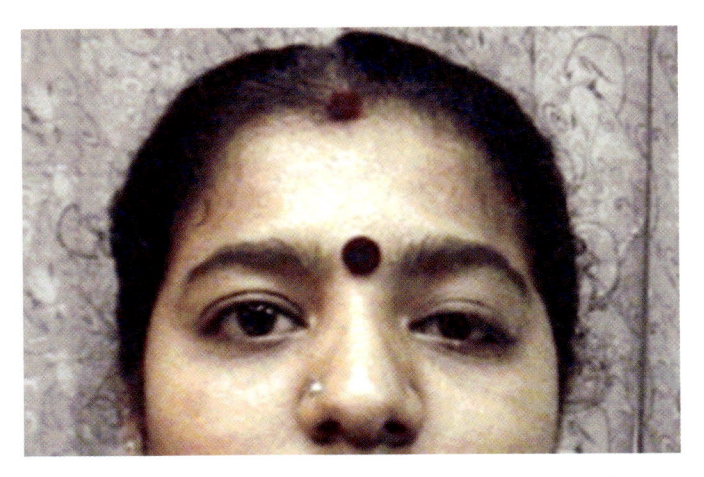

QUESTION 76

1. List the measurements that should be carried out in this patient.
2. Which two ocular tests are important in the pre-surgical workup?
3. In the Congenital form which associated ocular abnormalities can be seen?
4. On which test measurement does the type of surgical treatment to be carried out depend?
5. Which is the nerve that is misdirected in Marcus Gunn ptosis and What is the treatment of choice?

ANSWERS

1. The following measurements should be carried out in a case of ptosis: Marginal reflex distance (MRD), upper lid crease, levator function and palpebral fissure height.
2. Corneal reflex test and Bell's phenomenon test are important in the pre-surgical workup as the decision to operate should be deferred if these are abnormal.
3. The common abnormalities that are seen in congenital ptosis are: Defective elevation due to weakness of the superior rectus, blepharophimosis syndrome, Marcus Gunn phenomenon.
4. The amount and type of surgery to be done depends on the levator function test.
5. The mandibular division of the trigeminal nerve is thought to be misdirected to the levator muscle, i.e. the third nerve, in Marcus Gunn ptosis. The treatment of choice is frontalis suspension with or without levator disinsertion.

QUESTION 77

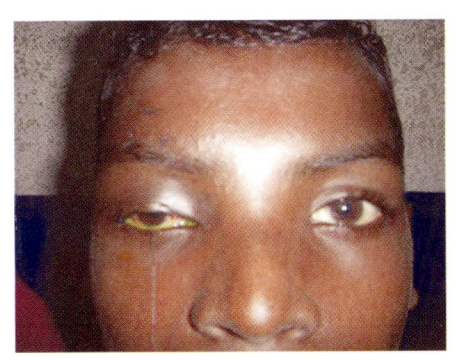

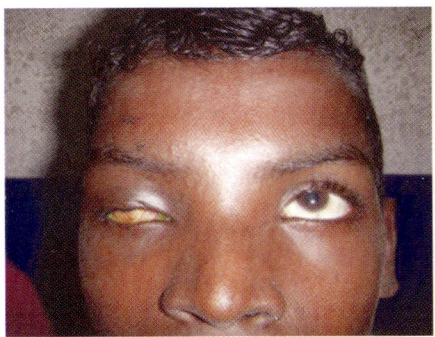

1. Identify the clinical condition.
2. What is the surgery done for the patient?
3. What are the four common materials used during this surgery?
4. Name the complications seen with silk and explain why?
5. Give the two common indications for carrying out this surgical procedure.

ANSWERS

1. This patient has postoperative ptosis with lagophthalmos.
2. He has undergone frontalis sling procedure.
3. The common material used are: Fascia lata, Mersilk, Ethibond, Polytetrafluoroethylene (PTFE).
4. Silk sutures are most commonly associated with suture granuloma and that is because silk remains non-integrated due to its property of poor biointegrity.
5. Frontalis sling is commonly done for: Congenital ptosis with poor levator function and for ptosis associated with Marcus Gunn jaw winking.

QUESTION 78

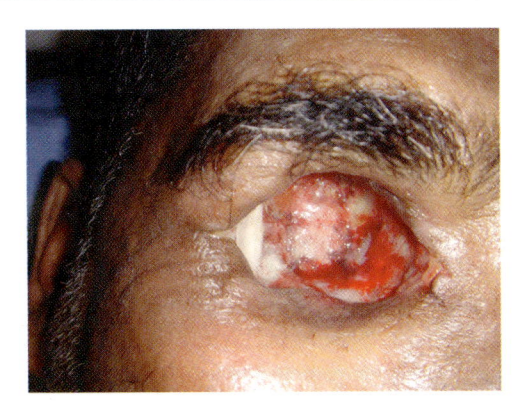

1. What surgical procedure has been done in this patient?
2. Name two common intraocular tumors that have to undergo this form of surgical procedure?
3. Which infection needs to be treated this way and in what kind of patients?
4. Classify this surgery based upon the amount of tissue removal.
5. What is the type that has been done here? Justify your answer.

ANSWERS

1. Exenteration has been done here.
2. Intraocular malignant melanoma and retinoblastoma with extraocular extension have to undergo exenteration.
3. Fungal orbital phycomycosis may need a total or a subtotal exenteration. It is commonly seen to such a severe grade in diabetics and immunocompromised patients.
4. Based upon the amount of tissue removal exenteration can be classified as total, subtotal, and extended.
5. A total exenteration has been done here, there is the removal of all the intraorbital soft tissue, including the periorbital, the underlying bare bony orbital wall is seen.

QUESTION 79

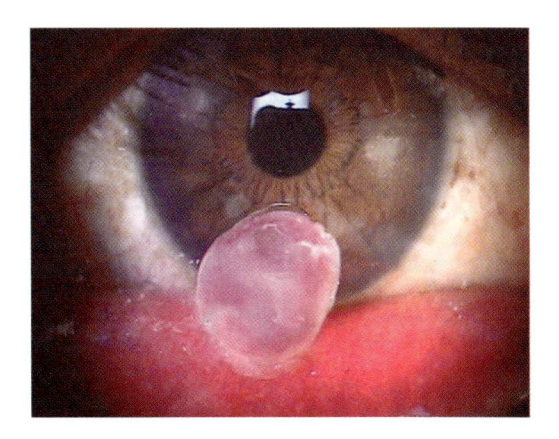

1. What does this patient have?
2. What is the differential diagnosis?
3. What will be the characteristic clinical finding in this patient?
4. How will you manage this patient?

ANSWERS

1. This patient has pyogenic granuloma.
2. The differential should be *retention cyst*.
3. The characteristic clinical finding will be presence of a pedunculated sessile nature of the granuloma.
4. This patient can be managed by surgical removal of the lesion with cautery of the underlying bed of conjunctiva.

QUESTION 80

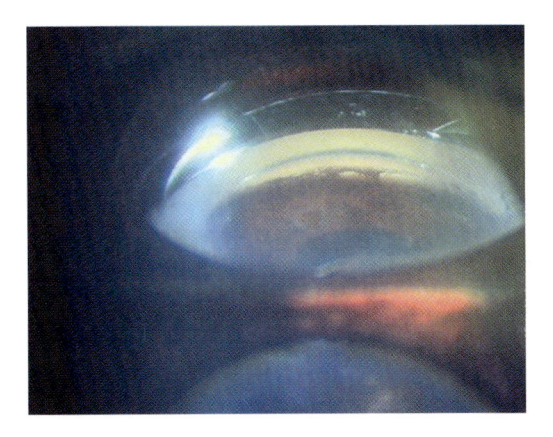

1. What is the abnormality seen at the angle?
2. What is the most common differential diagnosis? How will you differentiate the two?
3. What conditions give rise to pigment dispersion at the angle?
4. What is indentation gonioscopy? What is its role in this patient?
5. How will you manage this patient?

ANSWERS

1. There are open angles with peripheral anterior synechiae.
2. The most common differential is iris processes. They have extension beyond the trabecular meshwork, wheras the PAS do not cross the trabecular meshwork or Schwalbe's line. Normal angle structures can be seen behind the iris root, there is distortion of the angle structures in PAS. PAS tend to be irregular coarse in distribution and do not have a central core of blood vessel.
3. Pigment dispersion is seen in pigmentary glaucoma, post-uveitis eyes, post-trauma, exfoliation syndromes, post-intraocular surgery eyes commonly.
4. Gonio lenses of smaller diameter like the Zeiss lens are used where there is pressure applied to the central part if the cornea and this pushes the angles open as in case of appositional closure of the angle only. In case of PAS there is no opening of the angles seen.
5. The patient can be managed by doing a trabeculectomy – only when PAS is more than 180°.

QUESTION 81

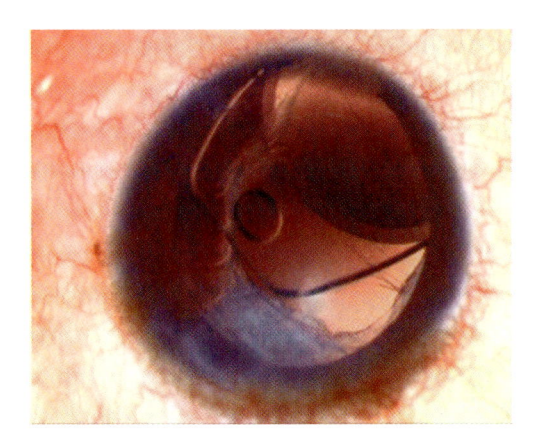

1. What does this patient have? What is the complication of surgery that has lead to the present state of the IOL?
2. What will this patient present with?
3. What are the primary causes of IOL displacement and secondary causes?
4. What will be the surgery planned for this patient?

ANSWERS

1. This patient has IOL subluxation or displacement. There is a posterior capsule rupture that is seen that would have caused this problem.
2. This patient will present with loss of BCVA, glare, halos, diplopia and pain in some cases.
3. Primary causes will be zonular dialysis and posterior capsular rupture on the table whereas the secondary causes are vigorous rubbing of the eyelids, trauma and capsular contracture that presents late.
4. The surgery that should be done should be explantation of this IOL with reimplantation using scleral fixated IOL or fibrin glue IOL in view of absent capsular bag.

QUESTION 82

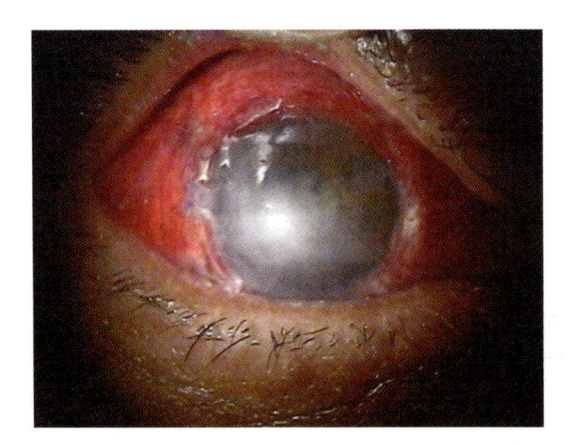

1. What condition does this patient have if an intraocular surgery had been done on him? What is the incidence?
2. What is the differential diagnosis?
3. Name the causes of late onset? In quieter eyes with less severe involvement. Why is it important to study the angles, what is the clinical test that is important?
4. What are the vision threatening complications? What will happen to the eye if left untreated?
5. How are intravitreal given and name the drugs?

ANSWERS

1. The patient has an endophthalmitis. The incidence is 0.15%.
2. The differential diagnosis is: TAS (toxic anterior segment), postoperative uveitis, retained lens material and vitreous hemorrhage.
3. The causes of late onset are: *P.acnes*, fungi like *Candida*, *Staph. epidermis* and Cornebacterium. It is important to study the angles so that a peripheral equatorial plaque is not missed and it is done by doing gonioscopy.
4. The vision threatening complications are macular ischemia, macular edema, retinal detachments and glaucoma. Untreated it causes pthisis and panophthalmitis with or without perforation.
5. Intravitreal should be given immediately after culture specimens have been obtained through pars plana from a site 4 mm in phakics and 3 mm in aphakics, after 0.2 to 0.3 ml has been aspirated, the drugs used are Ceftazidime and Vancomycin.

QUESTION 83

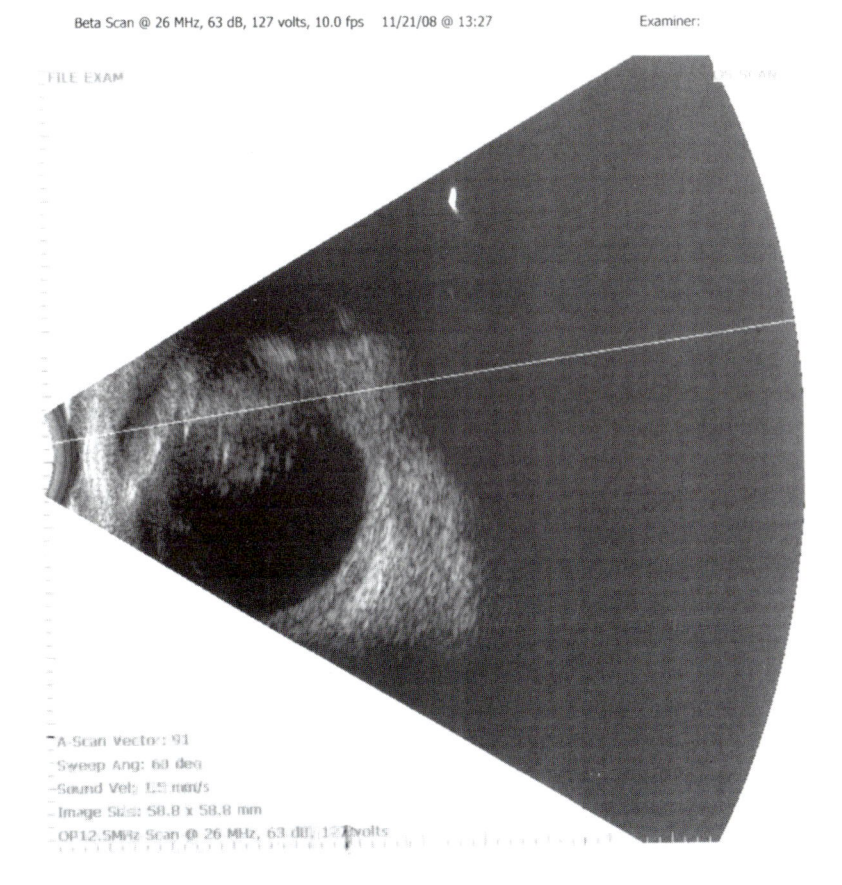

1. What does the B-scan picture show? Give common conditions that can be thought of?
2. What is the commonest primary intraocular malignancy? What is AFIP classification?
3. How will the tumor spread?
4. Under which conditions can the globe not be salvaged and will need an enucleation?

ANSWERS

1. The B-scan picture shows a acoustically hollow mass that is in the region of the uveal tissue. The common diagnosis can be ciliary body, Choroidal melanoma.
2. The commonest intraocular malignancy is choroidal melanoma, 90% of uveal melanomas are choroidal. The AFIP classification divides them into spindle cell and mixed that consists of spindle and epitheliod cells.
3. The modes of spread are via the vortex veins, via the scleral channels, through the RPE and Bruchs into the subretinal space and hematogenous spread to the liver, lungs, bones.
4. Large tumor involving the optic disc, extensive angle and ciliary body involvement, loss of all useful vision to the eye are cases where the globe cannot be salvaged.

QUESTION 84

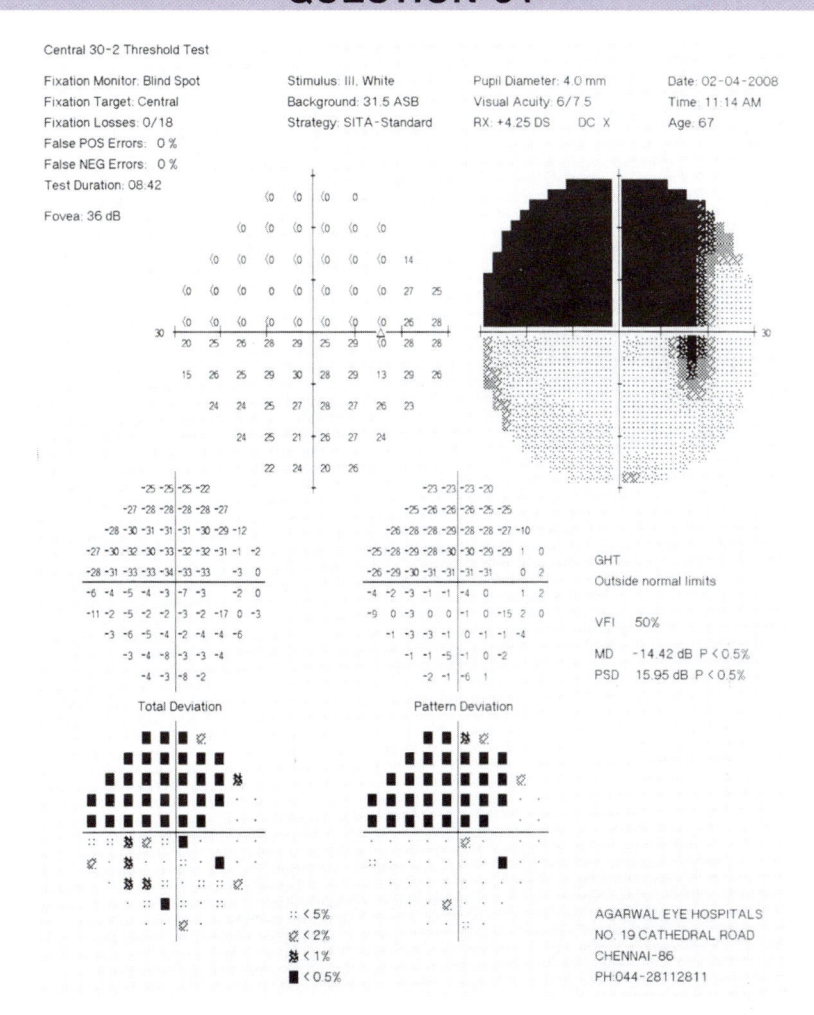

Central 30-2 Threshold Test

Fixation Monitor: Blind Spot
Fixation Target: Central
Fixation Losses: 0/18
False POS Errors: 0 %
False NEG Errors: 0 %
Test Duration: 08:42
Fovea: 36 dB

Stimulus: III, White
Background: 31.5 ASB
Strategy: SITA-Standard

Pupil Diameter: 4.0 mm
Visual Acuity: 6/7.5
RX: +4.25 DS   DC X

Date: 02-04-2008
Time: 11:14 AM
Age: 67

GHT
Outside normal limits

VFI   50%
MD   -14.42 dB P < 0.5%
PSD   15.95 dB P < 0.5%

Total Deviation   Pattern Deviation

:: < 5%
∅ < 2%
▨ < 1%
■ < 0.5%

AGARWAL EYE HOSPITALS
NO. 19 CATHEDRAL ROAD
CHENNAI-86
PH:044-28112811

1. What is this defect called? Name the condition causing it?
2. What are the vessels involved and what type of optic nerve head is predisposed to this condition?
3. When the other eye is involved, how do you call it?
4. What will be the FFA findings in the two varieties of the disease?
5. What should be the treatment in case of severe vision loss presentation and how is it hematologically and biochemistry monitored?

ANSWERS

1. The field defect shows altitudinal hemianopia. The condition that commonly causes it is AION.
2. The short posterior ciliary arteries are obstructed and discs with a small or a absent physiological cup are predisposed to obstruction.
3. Pseudo foster Kennedy syndrome occurs when the other eye is involved. Risk factors for the other eye involvement are: loss of vision in one eye and Diabetes mellitus.
4. The FFA picture in non-arteritic will show early and late disc hyperfluorescence and the arteritic AION will show absent choroidal fluorescence.
5. When the patient presents with severe vision loss the treatment should be intravenous methylprednisolone sodium succinate 1 gm daily and 80 mg oral steroid for 3 days, this is followed by a reduction. ESR and CRP are monitored for the therapy.

QUESTION 85

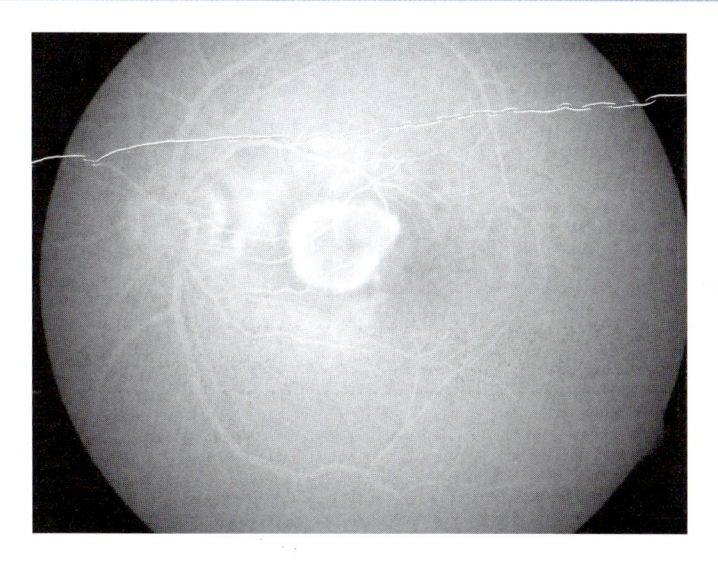

1. Which phase of FFA has this picture been taken? What is your diagnosis?
2. What will the different phases of the FFA show? How will the condition be classified on FFA?
3. Which condition will ICG be more useful?
4. What complications will occur in long standing cases?
5. Give the different modalities of treatment in this condition.

ANSWERS

1. This picture belongs to the venous phase. The patient has SRNVM.
2. The early phase of the FFA will show hyperfluorescence in a lacy pattern, venous phase shows hyperfluorescence well defined, late phase shows staining of the membrane. On FFA the SRNVM can be classified as classic, occult and fibrovascular PED.
3. ICG will be useful in occult poorly defined membranes, overlying hemorrhages, fluid and exudates.
4. The long standing cases can develop hemorrhagic PED, vitreous hemorrhages, disciform scarring and massive exudations.
5. The different modalities of treatment are PDT, intravitreal steroids, intravitreal anti-angiogenic factors and surgery that can be macular translocations, submacular surgery and pneumatic displacement surgeries.

QUESTION 86

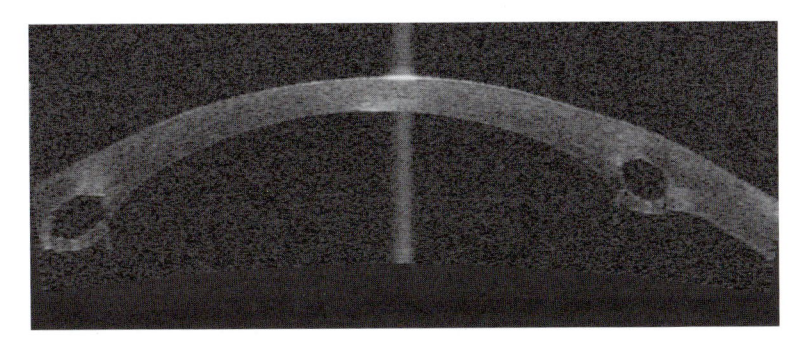

1. What procedure is performed for this patient?
2. Give two indications for this procedure.
3. Give one contraindication for this procedure.
4. What is it made of ?

ANSWERS

1. Patient has been implanted with corneal segment ring.
2. Low myopia, now used in keratoconus.
3. Corneal thickness less than 400 μm at the site of insertion.
4. PMMA.

QUESTION 87

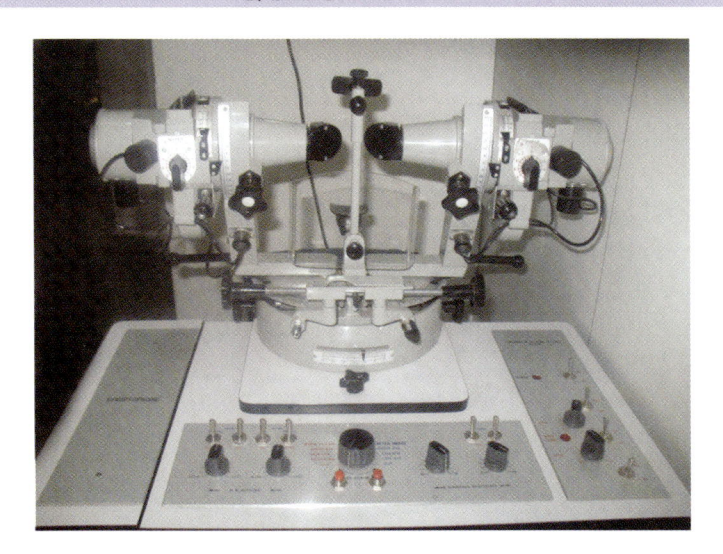

1. How is the objective angle measured?
2. What is the other name of this instrument?
3. What is the angle of anomaly if the subjective and objective angles are equal and what does this patient have?
4. What does the patient have if the angle of anomaly equals the objective angle and what is the subjective angle in such cases?
5. What types of slides are used while testing for ARC, angle kappa measurement?

ANSWERS

1. The objective angle is measured by flashing the light alternately in each eye along with movement of the arms until no further fixation movement of either eye is observed.
2. The other name of this instrument is major amblyoscope.
3. The object and subject angles are equal means that the angle of anomaly is zero and the patient has normal retinal correspondence.
4. If the objective angle equals the angle of anomaly then the patient has harmonious abnormal retinal correspondence and the subjective angle in such cases is zero.
5. While measuring ARC simultaneous macular perception slides are used, for angle kappa horizontal number and alphabet slide is used.

QUESTION 88

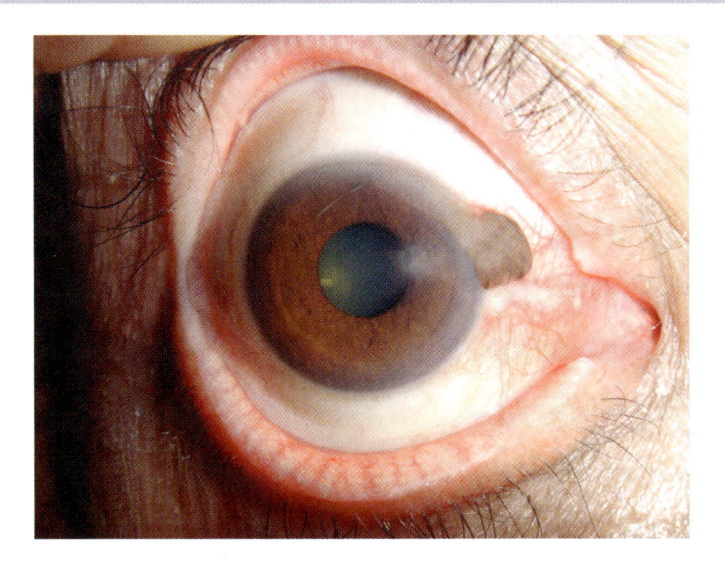

1. What is your clinical diagnosis? Give a common differential for this condition.
2. What is the typical appearance of a nonpigmented tumor called? What change in the appearance will cause suspicion of a malignant change?
3. What is the cause of pain in a ciliary body melanoma, list two?
4. What two clinical examinations are a must in this patient?
5. Give the ocular investigation of choice.

ANSWERS

1. This is a patient of conjunctival melanoma. A common differential diagnosis is ciliary body melanoma.
2. A nonpigmented tumor has a fish flesh appearance. The most suspicious change in appearance is the appearance of 1 or more nodules on the surface of a flat lesion.
3. Pain in a ciliary body melanoma is secondary to glaucoma and secondary to direct invasion of the long ciliary nerves.
4. This patient should undergo contact lens examination with a three mirror and also a trans-illumination test.
5. Ultrasound Biomicroscopy is the ocular investigation of choice.

QUESTION 89

STRATUS OCT
Retinal Thickness Report - 4.0.5 (0076)

SAROJINI, A

DOB: 11/18/1930, ID: 383150, Female

Scan Type: Macular Thickness Map OD
Scan Date: 11/18/2008
Scan Length: 6.0 mm

OCT Image

Fundus Image

Signal Strength (Max 10)	4
Analysis Confidence Low	
Retinal Thickness is	228 microns at A-scan 1
Caliper Length is	OFF

Normative Data is not available for Macular Thickness Map scan group

Thickness Chart

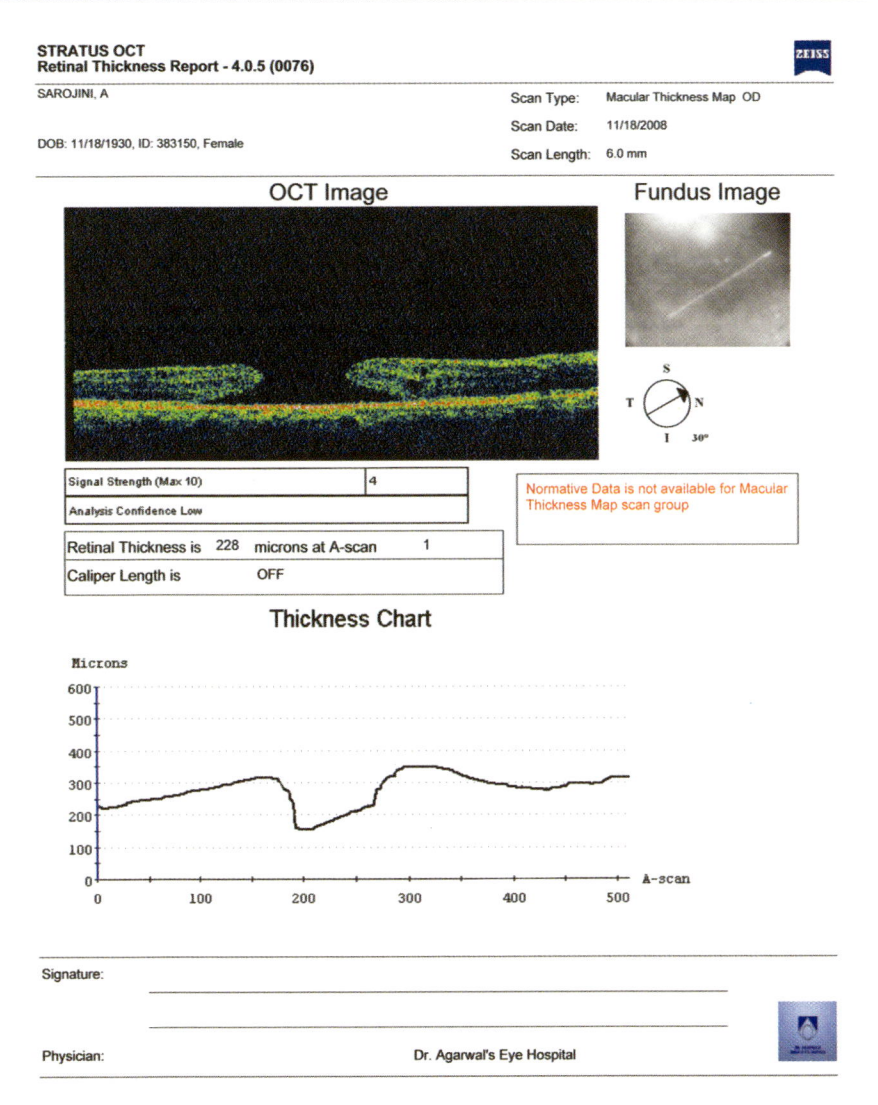

Signature: _____

Physician: Dr. Agarwal's Eye Hospital

1. Identify the disease? What stage of the diseases can this belong to?
2. What is the commonest cause and the most common pathogenic mechanism identified? Give the differential diagnosis on clinical examination of the patient.
3. What is Watske's sign? What will it be in this patient.
4. What are the risk factors of a premacular hole lesion progressing to a full thickness hole? Discuss with respect to VA on presentation FFA finding.

ANSWERS

1. This is an OCT macula that shows a full thickness macular hole. The stage can be stage 3 or stage 4.
2. The commonest cause is idiopathic, and the commonest pathogenesis is foveovitreal traction apart from being idiopathic. The differential diagnosis is CSR, CME, subfoveal exudates, serous RPE detachments.
3. Watske's sign is when there is a break in the slit lamp beam during slit lamp biomicroscopy using the 78 or 90D lens. The sign will be positive in these cases.
4. The risk factors are: Va: Less than 20/50 vision on presentation fundus finding: vitreomacular traction, and presence of partial PVD and presence of RPE changes on FFA.

QUESTION 90

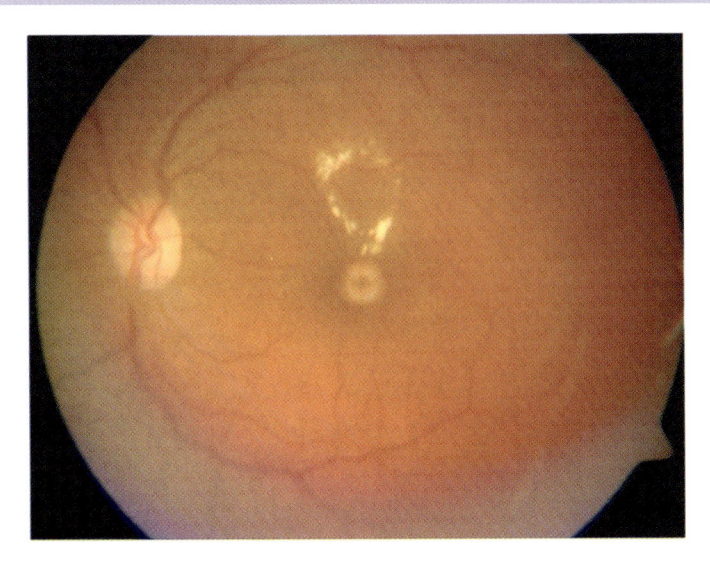

1. What will be your diagnosis on fundus picture?
2. What will be the criteria to call macular edema clinically significant?
3. What are the modalities of treatment in these patients?
4. What are the types of maculopathies associated?
5. What are the poor visual prognosis factors, with respect to
   - Systemic disease
   - Type of maculopathy
   - Two other macular features.

ANSWERS

1. This is a fundus picture of clinically significant macular edema with circinate retinopathy.
2. The following types of macular edema are clinically significant:
   - Retinal edema within 500 microns of the fovea
   - Hard exudates within 500 microns of the fovea associated with retinal thickening
   - Retinal edema larger than 1500 microns but a part of it is within 1 disc diameter of the foveal center.
3. The treatment can be laser that can be focal, grid pattern, intravitreal triamcinolone and intravitreal antiangiogenic factors.
4. The maculopathies associated with CSME are: Exudative, ischemic and edematous.
5. The indicators for poor prognosis are: systemic condition: Renal failure, maculopathy: ischemic maculopathy, Other macular features: lamellar macular hole and foveal exudates.

Section 4   189

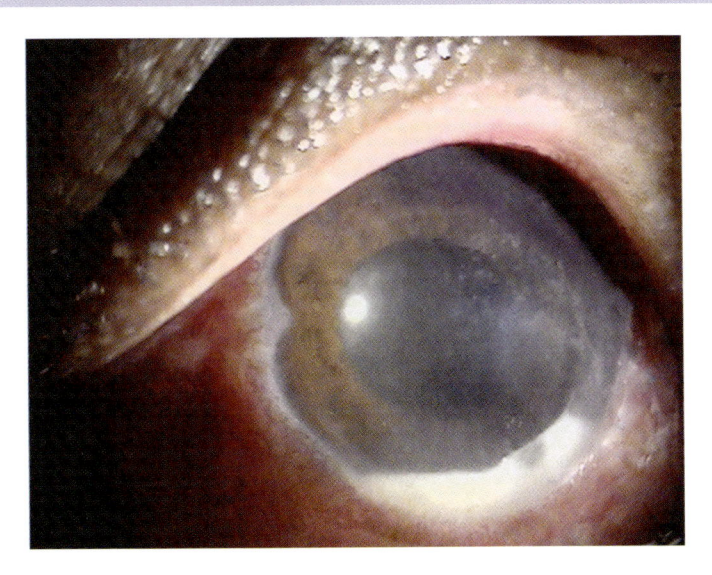

QUESTION 91

1. Which organism causes this condition, what is it called and what is its other name?
2. Name causes of pseudohypopyon? What are they also called?
3. Causes of hypopyon in quiet eyes.
4. What is inverse hypopyon?
5. How will you differentiate a fungal from a bacterial hypopyon?

ANSWERS

1. Pneumococcus causes this condition and it is called hypopyon corneal ulcer. The other name is serpiginous corneal ulcer.
2. The causes of pseudohypopyon are: Retinoblastoma, juvenile xanthogranuloma, leukemias and lymphomas. They are also called Masquerade syndromes.
3. The causes of hypopyon in quiet eyes are Behcets syndrome, and sterile hypopyon postoperative.
4. Inverse hypopyon is seen when silicone oil has been used for RD surgery and it comes to the anterior chamber.
5. Fungal hypopyon has convex upper border, hyphae seen, low mobility with head posture and yellow in color. Bacterial has a concave border, mobile with head posture, no hyphae seen and whitish in color.

QUESTION 92

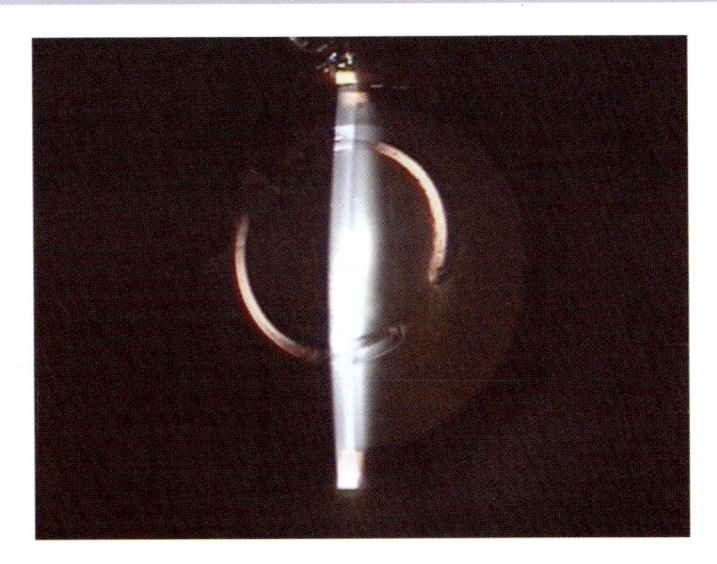

1. Identify the inserts in the photo. What will be the indication of placing a single ring only?
2. What should be the minimal corneal thickness to place them?
3. Name the indications where they should be done?
4. What will happens to the cornea – will it become more prolate or oblate after placing the rings?
5. What type of technology is this in treating refractive errors?
6. In a case of post-lasik ectasia what is taken into account while putting these segments – the residual bed or the total corneal thickness? Give your reasons.

ANSWERS

1. These are intracorneal ring segments that can be kerarings or intacs. A single ring is placed in cases of pellucid marginal degeneration.
2. The minimal corneal thickness should be 400 microns.
3. They are commonly done for treatment of keratoconus, pellucid marginal degeneration and spherical myopias.
4. The cornea becomes more prolate.
5. The technology is additive.
6. Post-lasik ectasia the residual bed thickness is taken as the rings are to be placed in the residual bed.

QUESTION 93

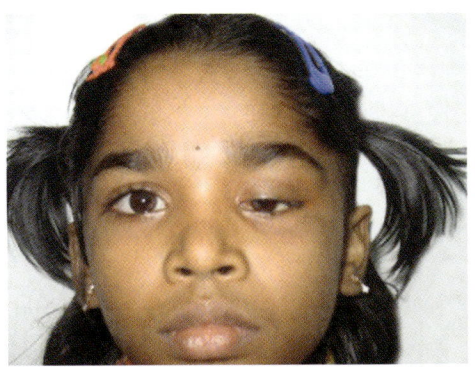

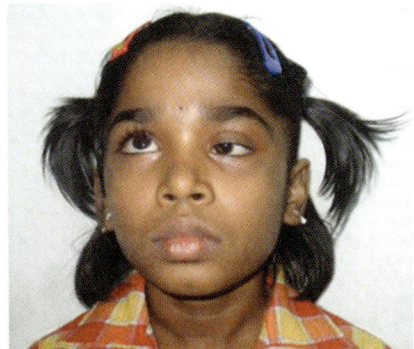

1. What is the clinical condition shown here?
2. Which are the muscles involved?
3. What will be the position of the eyes in primary position and on up gaze?
4. What will be the head posture of the child?
5. What % of patients have ptosis? What abnormal synkinesis is seen in such patients?

ANSWERS

1. Double elevator palsy is shown here.
2. The muscles involved are the inferior oblique and the superior rectus.
3. In primary position the eyes will be hypotropic and in up gaze the hypotropia will increase.
4. The child will have a chin up position in terms of head posture.
5. 50% of children will have ptosis and Marcus Gunn Jaw winking phenomenon is seen in these patients at times.

QUESTION 94

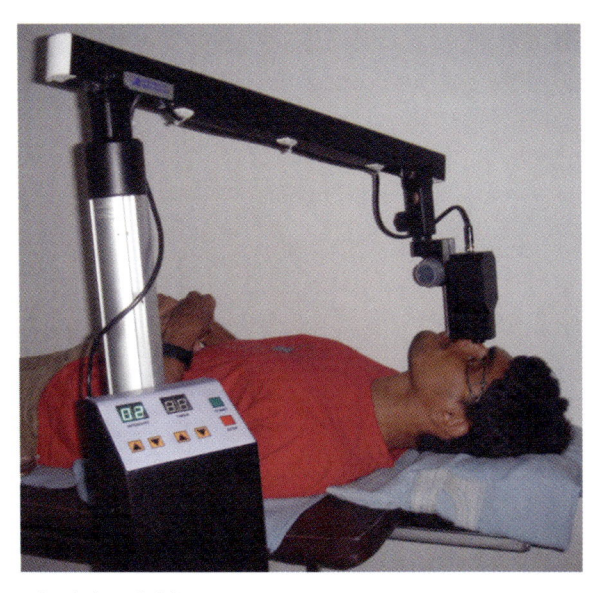

1. Name the principle of this treatment.
2. What are the indications of doing this treatment?
3. Which of the following increases the corneal thickness and resembles the same principle as the above mentioned treatment: Aging, diabetes, and hypertension?
4. What precaution should be taken before posting this patient for this treatment?

ANSWERS

1. The principle of the treatment is collagen cross-linking.
2. The indications are post-intracorneal rings in keratoconus, post-lasik ectasia.
3. Diabetes increases the corneal collagen cross-linking.
4. Before posting the patient the total thickness of the cornea should be measured and it should be more than 400 microns.

QUESTION 95

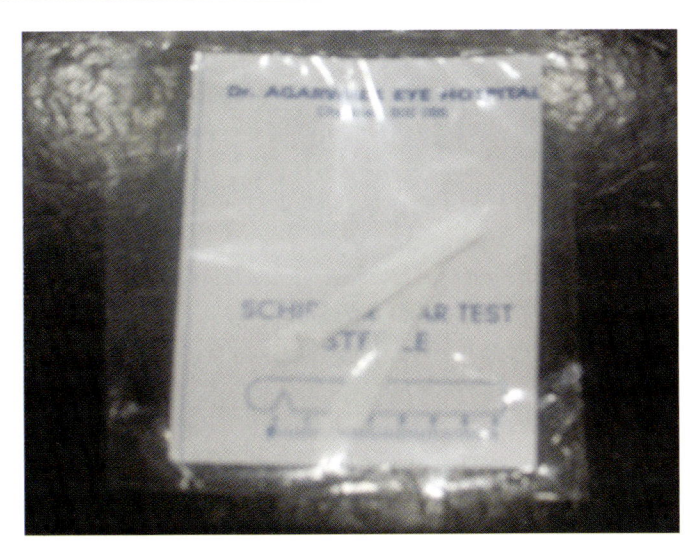

1. What are being shown here? What is their use and what are they made up of?
2. In test 2 what should be done? What does test 1 measure?
3. What is the normal value of tear wetting and what should be taken as the cut off point?
4. What are the other diagnostic tests done clinically? What should be done first TBUT or a Schirrmers? Why?
5. What are the methods to reduce tear drainage? State both the temporary and permanent methods.

ANSWERS

1. This is a Schirrmers strip. It is used in diagnosis of dry eye. It is made up of Whatmann no: 51 filter strip.
2. In test 2 anesthetic drops are put and the test 1 measures both the basal and reflex secretions.
3. The normal tear wetting of the strip is 15 mm anything below 5 mm is taken as impaired secretion.
4. Tear film meniscus height, debris, TBUT are the other clinical tests that can be performed. TBUT should be done first as a Schirrmers would create an artificial dry spot to appear at the point of its contact with the eye, thus falsely reducing the TBUT.
5. The temporary methods to reduce tear drainage are lacrimal plugs made of collagen; the permanent plugs are made of silicone. Then there is cautery of the punctum which is also practised to reduce the tear drainage.

QUESTION 96

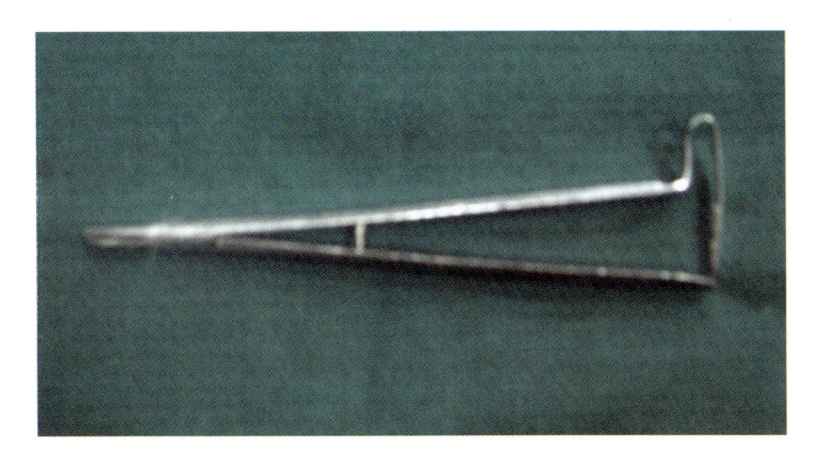

1. Identify this instrument.
2. List the uses of this instrument.
3. What is the blade used with this instrument?
4. Name another blade that is commonly used for making corneoscleral grooves.

ANSWERS

1. Barraquer blade breaker.
2. The uses are: Corneoscleral groove during cataract extraction surgery, stab incision into the AC while performing ECCE, stab side port entry while performing phacoemulsification.
3. The blade used are carbon razor blades.
4. Other blades in use are: Bard Parker blade no: 11 for entry and no: 15 for tunnel with a BP knife handle.

QUESTION 97

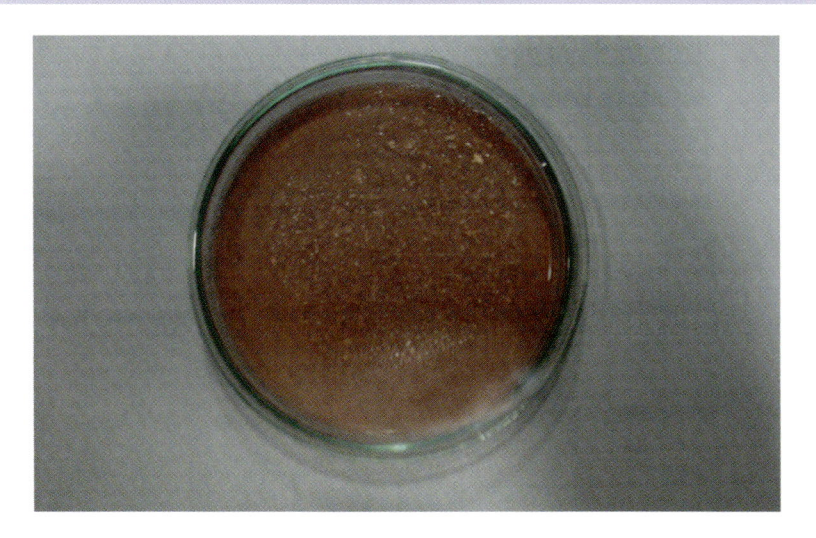

1. Identify the culture plate.
2. What organisms is it used for culture?
3. What is the colour of the colonies that grow on this media?
4. Name another media that can be used for the same organisms.

ANSWERS

1. This is a McConkey agar.
2. It is used for gram-negative organisms: *E.coli*, *Kliebsiella*, and *Pseudomonas*.
3. The colour of the colonies is pink.
4. Another media that can grow gram-negative organisms is: Nutrient agar.

QUESTION 98

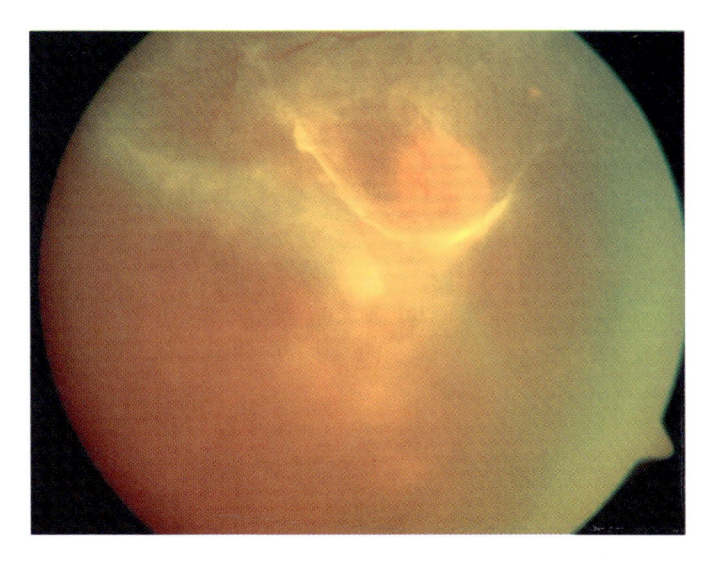

1. What does this picture show? Give your diagnosis.
2. Name the inflammatory causes of this picture.
3. What are the types of vitreoretinal tractions?
4. When should this patient be treated?
5. What is characteristic of tractional detachments in diabetic retinopathies and what are the poor prognostic factors?

ANSWERS

1. Tractional retinal detachment is the likely diagnosis. This picture shows the absence of retinal vessels, there is fibrovascular proliferation seen on the retinal surface with extension to the disc and pull on the underlying retina.
2. The inflammatory causes are: Eales diseases, cyclitic uveitis, toxoplasmosis and toxocariasis.
3. The types of Vitreoretinal tractions are: Anterioposterior, tangential, bridging tabletop and tent.
4. Tractional retinal detachments that should be treated are those which – involve the macula, associated with rhegmatogenous retinal detachments, associated with vitreous haemorrhages.
5. Diabetic tractional detachments remain confined to the posterior pole and rarely extend beyond the equator. Poor prognostic features are:
   – Long standing cases
   – Associated vitreous haemorrhages and
   – No previous PRP.

QUESTION 99

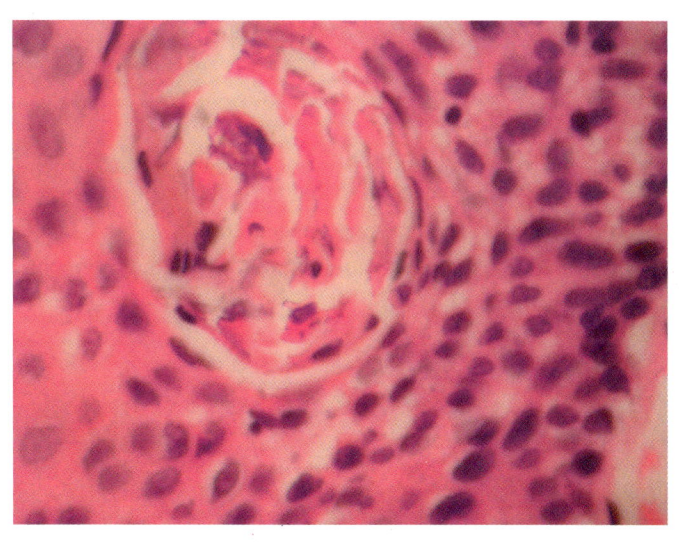

1. Give the diagnosis and describe the slide.
2. What are the conjunctival intraepithelial tumours (CIN).
3. What will be treatment in early and in advanced cases?
4. A long standing growth on the surface can be misdiagnosed as two other chronic conjunctivitis condition. Name there two conditions?

ANSWERS

1. The slide shows presence of onion peel nests characteristic of squamous neoplasia.
2. Tumours under CIN are: Bowen disease, carcinoma *in situ*, conjunctival dysplasia and intraepithelial epitheliomas.
3. The treatment involves local excision and cryo application at times. Advanced cases may need enucleation and even excenteration.
4. The common misdiagnosis is chronic conjunctivitis and atypical pterygium.

QUESTION 100

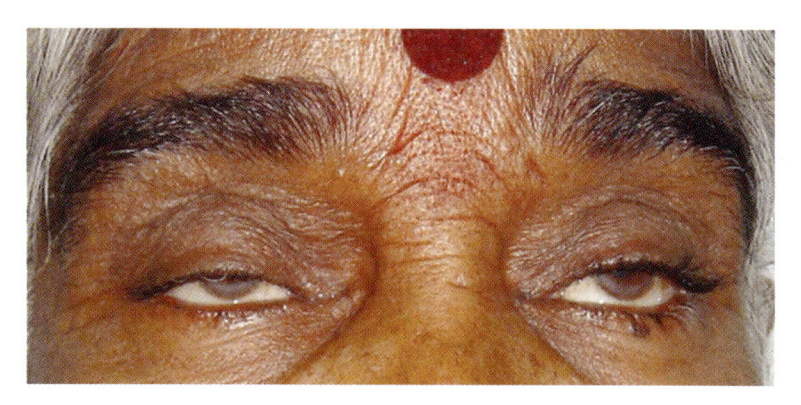

1. Give your diagnosis in this patient.
2. What are the other causes of similar clinical picture?
3. List the lid signs and gaze involvements that can be present in this patient.
4. What are the tests in the OPD that you will do to confirm this clinical condition?
5. Name the drugs exacerbating or causing this condition.

ANSWERS

1. This looks to be a patient of Myasthenia Gravis.
2. The other causes of bilateral lid drooping in adult are: thyroid, CPEO, myotonic dystrophy, orbital psuedotumour.
3. The lid signs are: lid fatigue, lid twitch sign of Cogan, ptosis. The gaze involvements are: gaze palsies, INO, gaze evoked nystagmus.
4. Tests that can be done are: ice test, lid fatigue test, sleep test, tensilon test and EMG.
5. Drugs causing myasthenia or exacerbating the condition are: penicillamine, aminoglycosides, quinidine and propanolol.

Section 5

Observation Stations

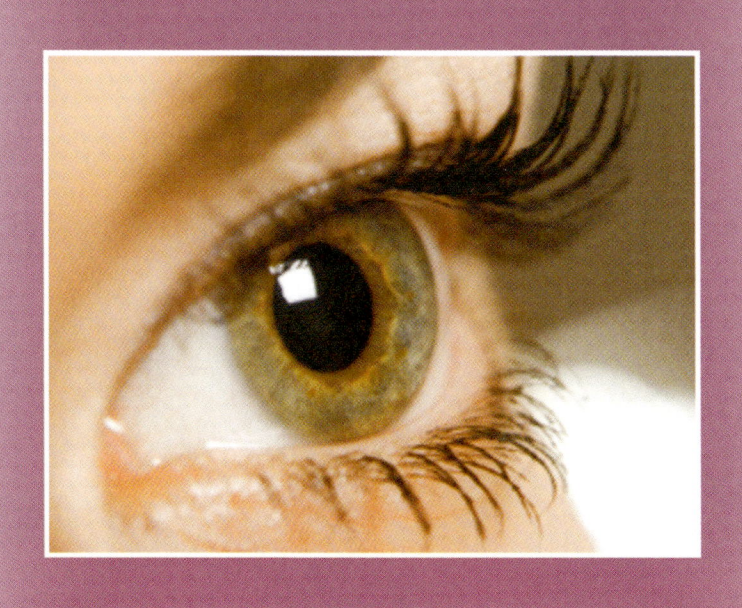

SLIT-LAMP EXAMINATION

Specular Reflection

- First step is to see that the eye pieces are set to zero or your glass power.
- Second step is to swing the illumination and the observation system to 90 degree apart.
- There should be high magnification.
- The width of the slit beam can be just less than the maximum and the height should be 3 mm.
- The patient is instructed to see straight ahead bisecting the angle formed between the illumination and observation systems.
- The specular reflection of the endothelial cells is obtained uniocularly only.

Retroillumination

- Can be done under any magnification. The slit lamp observation system and the illumination systems should be co-axial.
- The patient should be instructed to look straight ahead and the illumination system adjusted slowly to get the red glow from the fundus, in the pupil.
- By moving the joy stick towards the patient the cornea, iris, anterior lens surface and posterior lens surface and vitreous opacities can be identified against the red fundal glow.

Sclerotic Scatter

- Used to identify corneal opacities by using the principle of total internal reflection. Light is thrown on the temporal limbus in such a way that no illumination is visible. This is because the light is totally internally-reflected in between the anterior and posterior surfaces of the cornea. If an opacity is present in the cornea then it will be illuminated by the light beam travelling horizontally and internally within the cornea.

Applanation Tonometry

- Explain the procedure to the patient.
- First apply 2 or 4% xylocaine into the conjunctival sac.
- Check if the prism in the tonometer is set at 180.
- Adjust the reading in the tonometer body to read 1.
- Use low magnification.
- Swing the tonometer to in front of the slit-lamp and ensure that the prism is visible with one eye only and is in focus.

- Switch on the cobalt blue filter.
- Use maximum illumination.
- Switch off room lights.
- Gently applanate the cornea without exerting pressure on the lids.
- Instruct the patient not to blink.
- Take the reading by rotating the reading knob untill the mires overlap each other internally.
- Repeat the reading if too much or too little fluorescein is present with the right quantity of fluorescein.
- Apply a drop of antibiotic to the patient. Ask nurse to disinfect tonometer prism with sodium hypochlorite or isopropyl alcohol.

Gonioscopy

- Explain the procedure to the patient.
- Instill a drop of xylocaine 2 or 4% into the cul-de-sac.
- Inspect the gonioscope to see if its clean and which type is given- single mirror or 3 mirror.
- Dim the room lights.
- Ask patient to keep the chin in the slit-lamp and look straight ashed.
- Set low mag beam horizontal for examining the inferior and superior angle.
- Ask patient to look up.
- Apply viscoelastic or ky jelly in to the gonioscope and apply the gonioscope onto the lower sclera.
- Now ask the patient to gently look straight so that the gonioscope is on the cornea.
- Rotate the gonio mirror to 12 O'clock to see the inferior angle.
- Be careful to see that the illumination does not fall on the pupil as it will constrict the pupil and result in an opening up of the narrow angle.
- Record which is the posterior most structure you can see for example cilliary body grade 4, scleral spur grade 3, trabecular meshwork grade 2 and schwalbes line grade 1.
- Look for abnormal pigmentation, cells, debris, pseudoexfoliation material, peripheral anterior synechiae, peripheral iridotomy, cyclodialysis cleft and internal ostium of a trabeculectomy.
- Rotate the mirror 360° gently without letting air bubbles to get entrapped in between the gonioscope and the cornea. Record your findings.
- Gently remove the gonioscope from the eye by asking the patient to look up and tilting the upper end of the gonioscope outwards.
- Clean the eye with a cotton instill a drop of antibiotic into the eye. Clean the gonioscope.

Retinoscopy

- Greet the patient and explain the procedure.
- Check for dilatation of pupil and cycloplegia.
- Make the patient sit properly and choose your working distance as 1/2 or 2/3 meter.
- Put on the trial frame on the patient. Ask the patient to fixate on the 6/60 letter on the chart.
- Start with the right eye of the patient sit to the left of the patient and use your right eye.
- Hold the retinoscope with your right hand with the thumb on the sleeve to make it vertical or horizontal. Make sure the illumination is adequate and that the plane mirror is selected.
- Move the streak horizontally twice to check movement. Then rotate it vertically with your thumb and move the retinoscope by moving your wrist not your entire hand or body.
- Select the appropriate spherical lens from the trial frame to neutralise the reflex. Chose the appropriate power, for example a slow moving with reflex in an aphake start with +9.0.
- Chose the next lenses systematically going for higher powers until neutralisation is reached.
- Record your horizontal and vertical readings as the power cross.
- Repeat for the other eye by sitting at the right side of the patient for his left eye and use your left eye for the retinoscopy. Remember to wear your spectacle correction while doing retinoscopy.

Subjective Refraction

- Explain the procedure to the patient.
- Ask which language the patient can read well.
- Note the retinoscopy in the power cross form and the working distance.
- Write the new power cross after subtracting the working distance.
- Now start the subjective refraction by choosing the appropriate sphere and cylinder. First find the axis of the cylinder, then refine the cylinder power with a Jackson's cross cylinder.
- Remember to fog the patient if you are dealing with a hypermetrope. That is start with higher plus lenses and reduce to get better vision. In case of minus powers start with smaller power then increase the power untill you get the final value.
- Finally, do a duochrome test to confirm your correction.
- If patient is undilated check his near vision.